Current Practices in Ophthalmology

Series Editor

Parul Ichhpujani
Department of Ophthalmology
Government Medical College and Hospital
Chandigarh, India

T0073198

This series of highly organized and uniform handbooks aims to cover the latest clinically relevant developments in ophthalmology. In the wake of rapidly evolving innovations in the field of basic research, pharmacology, surgical techniques and imaging devices for the management of ophthalmic disorders, it is extremely important to invest in books that help you stay updated. These handbooks are designed to bridge the gap between journals and standard texts providing reviews on advances that are now part of mainstream clinical practice. Meant for residents, fellows-in-training, generalist ophthalmologists and specialists alike, each volume under this series covers current perspectives on relevant topics and meets the CME requirements as a go-to reference guide. Supervised and reviewed by a subject expert, chapters in each volume provide leading-edge information most relevant and useful for clinical ophthalmologists. This series is also useful for residents and fellows training in various subspecialties of ophthalmology, who can read these books while at work or during emergency duties. Additionally, these handbooks can aid in preparing for clinical case discussions at various forums and examinations.

More information about this series at http://www.springer.com/series/15743

Adit Gupta • Prerana Tahiliani

Editors

Orbit and Oculoplastics

Newer Trends

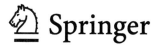 Springer

Editors
Adit Gupta
Mumbai Eye Plastic Surgery
Mumbai
Maharashtra
India

Prerana Tahiliani
Mumbai Eye Plastic Surgery
Mumbai
Maharashtra
India

ISSN 2523-3807   ISSN 2523-3815   (electronic)
Current Practices in Ophthalmology
ISBN 978-981-13-8540-7   ISBN 978-981-13-8538-4   (eBook)
https://doi.org/10.1007/978-981-13-8538-4

This Springer imprint is published by the registered company Springer Nature Singapore Pte Ltd.
The registered company address is: 152 Beach Road, #21-01/04 Gateway East, Singapore 189721, Singapore

Foreword

When I did my fellowship training with Dr. Norman Shorr 30 years ago, I remember thinking that oculoplastic and orbital surgery was so advanced that it had pretty much reached an apex, and it would be difficult to make any significant further advances in the field. Just in case the lesson of how wrong I was is not obvious, simply glance at the table of contents of the excellent handbook that Adit and Prerana have put together: the field has blossomed in extraordinary fashion over the past 30 years, and our ability to help patients with difficult eyelid, lacrimal and orbital disease is amazing.

I am most proud to congratulate the editors: they have tapped some of the best experts in the world to present cutting-edge information on an excellent choice of practical topics. Each chapter covers an important and challenging aspect of our discipline, and each of these areas has benefited from significant advances in both surgical and non-surgical management. I am hopeful that the readers will be able to apply this knowledge to their own patients.

Most of all, I hope that the readers are personally motivated to further evolve the Discipline of Ophthalmology. Whether you are a professor at a busy urban university, or a solo practitioner in a small town, you have the ability to discover new things and invent better ways to help our patients. Hopefully the ideas in this textbook, and the passion and talent of the authors and editors of the book, will inspire you in your own journey.

And especially if you are young, brace yourself: medicine and science are evolving at increasing speed, and the advances that you will see in your career will surely take your breath away.

Robert Alan Goldberg
UCLA Stein Eye Institute
Los Angeles, CA, USA

Contents

About the Editors

Adit Gupta is a double fellowship trained Oculofacial Plastic Surgeon. Over the past 8 years, he has performed several procedures for the cosmetic, structural, and functional rehabilitation of the eyelids and lacrimal region in India and the USA. He completed his MD in Ophthalmology at the Advanced Eye Centre, PGI Chandigarh, after which he completed his Oculoplasty fellowship at the LV Prasad Eye Institute in Hyderabad. He pursued further training for his second international fellowship (in orbitofacial cosmetic surgery) at the UCLA Stein Eye Institute, Los Angeles, California. Dr. Gupta's current focus is on cosmetic eyelid surgeries, complicated orbital surgeries, and rehabilitation of patients with thyroid eye disease. Apart from clinical work, he is actively involved in researching, developing, and teaching minimally invasive techniques for orbital and cosmetic surgeries.

Prerana Tahiliani is the founder of Mumbai Eye Plastic Surgery, a dedicated ophthalmic plastic surgery centre in the city of Mumbai. She completed her postgraduate training at Sri Sankaradeva Nethralaya, Guwahati, followed by a fellowship in Ophthalmic Plastic Surgery and Ocular Oncology at the LV Prasad Eye Institute, Hyderabad. During her time at LV Prasad, she developed a keen interest in ocular oncology and ophthalmic plastic surgery. She followed this up with research stays at the UCLA, CHLA, Los Angeles, and the Jules Gonin Eye Institute in Lausanne. Her current focus is on ocular oncology, cosmetic eyelid surgeries, and nonsurgical rejuvenation of the face. She is an active researcher and avid teacher who enjoys encouraging the younger generation to take up this subspecialty.

The Role of Photography in Oculofacial Aesthetics

1

Akshay Gopinathan Nair

In order to obtain a photograph that provides genuine information, strict uniformity and standardization are needed and this is best accomplished by using a simple and consistent scheme for photography [1]. Photographic images in oculofacial plastic surgery play a critical role not only in photo-documentation but also for preoperative planning, patient education, as well as medico-legal and insurance purposes. Additionally, consistent and high-quality photographs present the best opportunity for critical self-education and self-assessment [2, 3]. This chapter will discuss the basic photography techniques that are relevant to oculofacial surgery and a few pointers on how to achieve standardization.

Standardization is extremely important in facial photography because even subtle or minor changes in patient positioning and illumination of facial expressions during photo documentation for surgical procedures can cause the before and after procedure photos to be different and thereby leading to a sub-optimal comparison. All parameters in the photographs should remain the same—by doing so, one can ensure that the only thing that changes over time is the effect of the treatment—surgical or otherwise (Fig. 1.1).

Consent

A comprehensive informed consent that has been read, verified and signed by the patient is extremely essential before photography. It should explicitly state that the photographs are a part of the patient's medical records and that the photographs may be used for presentations, lectures and publications. The consent must be a part of

A. G. Nair (✉)
Ophthalmic Plastic Surgery and Ocular Oncology Services,
Advanced Eye Hospital and Institute, Navi Mumbai, Maharashtra, India

Ophthalmic Plastic Surgery and Ocular Oncology Services, Aditya Jyot Eye Hospital,
Mumbai, Maharashtra, India

© Springer Nature Singapore Pte Ltd. 2019   1
A. Gupta, P. Tahiliani (eds.), *Orbit and Oculoplastics*, Current Practices in
Ophthalmology, https://doi.org/10.1007/978-981-13-8538-4_1

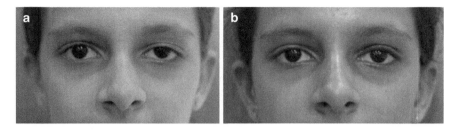

Fig. 1.1 A clinical photograph of a patient with congenital ptosis (**a**) and 1 week following the surgery with a well-corrected eyelid contour (**b**). The magnification, patient positioning and illumination in both photos are consistent, allowing the viewer to make an objective comparison

the medical records of the patient—physical or electronic. However, whenever reproduced in publications or book chapters, the clinician must take care that whenever possible, cropping or obscuring must be done such that the patient's identity is not revealed through the photographs. Furthermore, healthcare professionals must understand that in some cases, patients may not want to be photographed and they may not consent for the same—this should not change the standard or quality of care given [3].

Patient Preparation

The patient's hair must be tucked behind the ears or tied in such a way that it does not obscure the facial anatomy or the area of interest. Make-up and jewellery must be avoided at all costs as it can be distracting. Any garments or accessories such as head-scarves that interfere with the required pose or the visibility of the area to be photographed must be removed/repositioned [3].

Which camera should one choose for the clinic?

1. **Digital single lens reflex camera:** A digital single lens reflex (D-SLR) camera is an ideal camera for medical photography. This is primarily because these D-SLR cameras allow the user to customize the settings and modifying the three most important variables in photography, namely aperture, exposure and shutter speed.

   Aperture: Aperture refers to the opening of a lens's diaphragm through which the light passes. The aperture stop of the lens can be adjusted to control the amount of light reaching the film or image sensor.

   In combination with variation of shutter speed, the aperture size regulates the film's or image sensor's light exposure. Aperture sizes are measured by f-stops. A high f-stop (e.g. f-22) implies that the aperture hole is very small, and on the other hand, a low f-stop (e.g. f-1.8) indicates that the aperture is wide open thus allowing in more light.

   Shutter: The shutter is a small 'curtain' in the camera that quickly shuts over the image sensor of the camera and allows light to shine onto the sensor for just

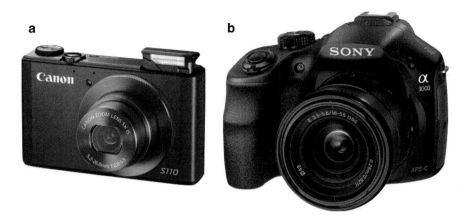

Fig. 1.2 A simple 'point and shoot' camera (**a**) and the larger bulkier D-SLR camera (**b**)

a fraction of a second [3]. The longer the shutter time, the brighter the picture since more light is gathered. On the other hand, a dark picture can be accounted by a very small shutter time as light touches the imaging sensor for a tiny fraction of a second. The combination of aperture and shutter speed can be manipulated to produce bright crisp photos [4].

2. **'Point-and-shoot' camera:** The small, compact 'point-and-shoot' cameras allow limited manipulation of the parameters, thereby making standardization and reproduction of the photographs difficult. These cameras click images in 'auto' mode and adjust the parameters on the basis of the ambient surrounding lighting.

3. **'Prosumer' camera:** In D-SLR cameras, the user can change the lens that can be attached to the body of the camera as opposed to point-and-shoot cameras, which usually have a fixed lens (Fig. 1.2) [3, 4]. In the past few years, a crossover breed of cameras is also available—called 'prosumer camera', wherein prosumer implies a professional consumer. These cameras are essentially easy to use point-and-shoot with some advanced features of D-SLRs [3]. While choosing a lens, a 90–105 mm lens should be preferred to avoid any image distortion and allow for a comfortable working distance [2].

Lighting and Background

Hard lighting: In case of bright lights, the resultant illumination would be considered hard lighting because of the harsh shadows it creates.

Soft lighting: Soft light results in shadows with soft edges or no defined edges at all. Using a single, camera mounted flash can produce a very bright flash of light which blanches finer details on the skin and also washes out the skin colour and tone [5]. When clicking for facial rejuvenation and resurfacing procedures, one must avoid direct flash. Hence, in order to capture facial redness and pigmentation, one must use soft and diffused light that is devoid of sharp lines and shadows.

Diffuse illumination can be obtained by using 'soft boxes' (Fig. 1.3) or 'speedlights' (Fig. 1.4) which can be fixed atop DSLR cameras. As it has been emphasized previously, the photographer has to ensure that the illumination used is the same in all photographs. The preferred background for all photos should be a non-reflective surface of a neutral colour—such as blue, white or grey. A pre-designated photography area should be used for patient photography such that uniformity is maintained.

Fig. 1.3 A soft light typically creates even and diffused light by transmitting light through some scattering material or surface or by reflecting light off a second surface to diffuse the light

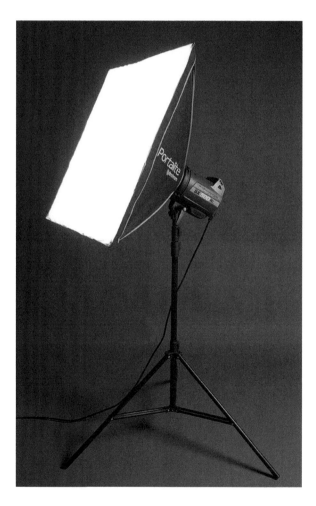

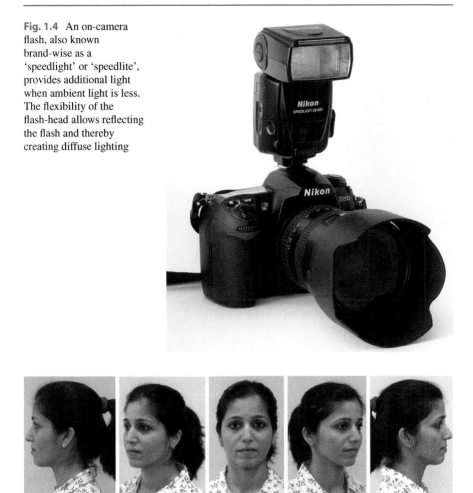

Fig. 1.4 An on-camera flash, also known brand-wise as a 'speedlight' or 'speedlite', provides additional light when ambient light is less. The flexibility of the flash-head allows reflecting the flash and thereby creating diffuse lighting

Fig. 1.5 The set of five photographs includes the frontal view, two lateral and two oblique views

Patient Positioning

The absolute essential photographs for any patient who visits a plastic surgeon/ cosmetic dermatologist for any facial issue are a set of five photographs consisting of the frontal view, two oblique views and two lateral views. This set of five photographs is a must at every consultation (Fig. 1.5) [2, 3]. The patients are asked to sit on a stool or a chair at least a foot in front of the background with their hands on their knees and a neutral expression on the face.

1. *Reference planes:*
   - *Frankfurt plane:* The Frankfort plane helps to standardize the horizontal plane in lateral, oblique and frontal views (Fig. 1.6). This plane is established

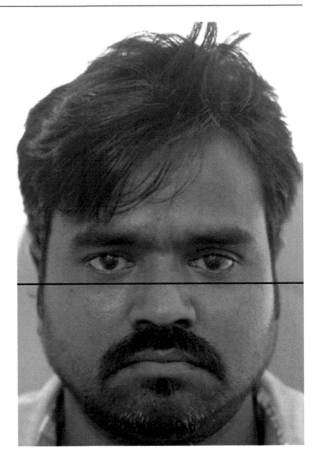

Fig. 1.6 Note the 'Frankfurt Plane' passing between the top of the tragus (or external auditory canal) and the infraorbital rim. This plane/line must be horizontal

by a line between the top of the tragus (or external auditory canal) and the infraorbital rim. In some cases, it might be difficult to mark the infraorbital rim as it is a bony landmark and not always easily found as a surface landmark. More practically, the rim may be palpated before positioning.

- *Midsagittal plane:* The midsagittal plane also helps to align the head position in frontal views [3, 4, 6].

2. *Views:*
   - *Frontal view:* A 'true' frontal view is achieved when both the ears are seen in the frontal photograph. The correct frontal view should have the canthi or tragi at the same horizontal level [6].
   - *Oblique view:* For the oblique views, the patient's body is turned 45° towards the photographer and he/she is asked to look ahead and only a narrow strip of cheek is seen behind the nose. The patient looks ahead and the Frankfurt plane must be held horizontal. While clicking the oblique view, one should not ask the patient to turn his/her face 45°, instead the whole body must be turned 45° to the photographer and photographs must be captured on both sides such that the right and the left sides.

- *Lateral view:* In lateral view photographs, the patient's head must face forward with the patient looking straight ahead. This is because even a small amount of head retrusion or neck flexion can greatly enhance the effect of sub-mental fat/jowl line. Conversely, neck extension or head protrusion can make the jowl line look better and reduce the appearance of submental soft tissue, thus simulating a successful lower facial rejuvenation [6].

3. *Specific views for specific conditions:* As Roberts et al. have mentioned, 'patients often retain more of what they see and less of what they hear' [7]. This holds true, especially, in the practice of aesthetic medicine, where it is extremely important to document the pre-procedural condition such that an accurate comparison can be made later.

   - *Proptosis:* Proptosis can be well highlighted through clinical photographs. A worm's eye view or a bird's eye view best highlights the severity of proptosis. A worm's eye view is more convenient and reproducible (Fig. 1.7). Here, the head is bent backward so as to align the nasal tip with brows on a horizontal plane. The camera should focus on the corneas.

   - *Ptosis:* For ptosis, in addition to the frontal view photograph, two separate photographs are shot with both eyes looking straight: one with frontalis over action (if present) followed by one without the frontalis over action. These are followed by one where the subject is looking down to document any preoperative downgaze lid lag and the last photograph with the eyes closed and the brow relaxed to document preoperative lagophthalmos, if present [4].

   - *Forehead lines, frown lines and crow's feet:* These are common conditions that are treated using botulinum toxin. To highlight these, specific photographs should be taken. For the forehead wrinkles, one photograph should be taken while asking the patient to elevate his/her eyebrows. The frontalis action makes the horizontal creases prominent. This photograph of the entire face is taken in the frontal view. Crow's feet appear over time from repeated contraction of the lateral portion of the orbicularis oculi. These features are highlighted best in the oblique and the lateral views. The patient should be asked to smile to make the crow's feet prominent. Oftentimes, the patient may not smile 'completely' and may require to be coaxed into smiling excessively to induce the appearance of crow's feet and orbicularis rolls (which

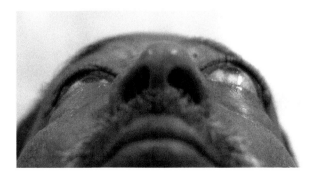

Fig. 1.7 The worm's eye view. Note that the tip of the nose is in line with the eyebrows and the camera is focused on the corneas with the patient looking straight ahead

cause the palpebral aperture to appear smaller on smiling) [3, 4]. This is one of the scenarios where lighting plays an extremely important role. Bright flash photography can bleach out the fine wrinkles giving a false 'smooth appearance', and they may not appear prominent in the photos. In cases of the use of botulinum toxin in the masseter for cases of masseter hypertrophy or for facial or jawline reshaping, the colour of the background and patient positioning play important roles in highlighting the outline of the masseter in the frontal view. The colour of the background should be in contrast to the patient's skin colour such that the face easily offsets against the background and the outline is easily appreciated [3]. The patient is asked to frown using his/her eyebrows. The forehead and eyebrows, which are the areas of interest, may be cropped later. In all cases, the frontal and the oblique views are supposed to include the head and neck, up to the jugular incisures including the platysmal bands.

- *Lid masses:* For lid masses, moles and other flat or pigmented lesions, the 'macro' mode may be used. Macro photography is extreme close-up photography and macro lenses allow the photographer to focus closer to the subjects than conventional optics, which lets one capture even finer details with greater clarity (Fig. 1.8).

Storage and Cataloguing

Securely storing, archiving and classifying patient photographs is an important aspect of clinical photography without which, it is difficult to retrieve photographs for comparisons. Many archival services are available, namely Cumulus (by Canto), which offers online (cloud-based) archiving. Other photography portfolio management software packages are PhotoDirector, ACDSee and Magix Photo Manager [3].

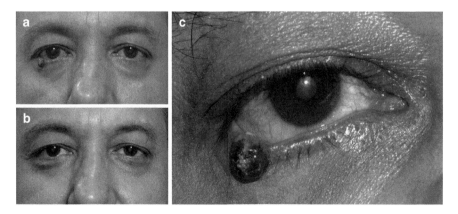

Fig. 1.8 The before (**a**) and after (**b**) surgery photos of a patient with a lower lid sebaceous gland carcinoma. (**c**) Macro-mode photo showing the details of the tumour well—ulceration, bleeding and the yellowish nodular component

The photographer can categorize date-wise; create separate folders for every patient and add customized keywords—based on the diagnosis. Also, the original photos must also be stored on hard-drives that are securely kept.

Unless there is no alternative, phones should not be used as a substitute for clinical photography. The use of smartphones to shoot clinical photographs of patients especially facial photographs is not encouraged as usual practice as they cannot replace the high resolution and reproducibility that cameras have. Poor screen resolution, lens induced distortion and graining in poor lighting are the flaws of mobile photography that cannot be overcome. Additionally, photographs, if stored on the phone, can be sent to other recipients. This transmission is irreversible, and the images once transmitted are permanently stored in the archives of the recipients—the further usage of which, the original sender has no control over [8, 9].

To summarize, the clinician must ensure patient consent is obtained before photography. One must employ a simple and systematic approach to clinical photography that guarantees optimal photographic results through standardized views for specific conditions. The key is in maintaining uniformity. In addition, responsible and safe storage go a long way in safeguarding the interests of the patient and the surgeon [3, 4].

Disclosures Consultant, HelpMeSee Inc., New York; USA.

Disclaimer All patient photographs in this chapter have been used after obtaining a written informed consent from the patients.

References

1. Becker DG, Tardy ME Jr. Standardized photography in facial plastic surgery: pearls and pitfalls. Facial Plast Surg. 1999;15(2):93–9.
2. Thomas JR, Tardy ME Jr, Przekop H. Uniform photographic documentation in facial plastic surgery. Otolaryngol Clin N Am. 1980;13(2):367–81.
3. Nair AG, Santhanam A. Clinical photography for periorbital and facial aesthetic practice. J Cutan Aesthet Surg. 2016;9(2):115–21.
4. Mukherjee B, Nair AG. Principles and practice of external digital photography in ophthalmology. Indian J Ophthalmol. 2012;60(2):119–25.
5. Shah AR, Dayan SH, Hamilton GS. Pitfalls of photography for facial resurfacing and rejuvenation procedures. Facial Plast Surg. 2005;21(2):154–61.
6. Sommer DD, Mendelsohn M. Pitfalls of nonstandardized photography in facial plastic surgery patients. Plast Reconstr Surg. 2004;114:10–4.
7. Roberts J, Roberts W. BOTOX and photography. Dent Today. 2010;29(6):120–1.
8. Nair AG, Potdar NA, Dadia A, Aulakh S, et al. Patient perceptions regarding the use of smart devices for medical photography: results of a patient-based survey. Int Ophthalmol. 2019;39(4):783–9. https://doi.org/10.1007/s10792-018-0878-2.
9. Natarajan S, Nair AG. Outsmarted by the smartphone! Indian J Ophthalmol. 2015;63:757–8.

Orbital Vascular Malformations: Current Concepts

2

Sathyadeepak Ramesh and Daniel Rootman

Introduction

Vascular anomalies are thought to be congenital lesions, although they can present across all age ranges. Diversity in the physiologic and anatomic characteristics of such lesions leads to a wide array of clinical presentations. Understanding the cellular and flow characteristics of vascular malformations, as well as their appropriate nomenclature, allows for systematic study and appropriate application of management techniques. In this chapter, we provide an overview of current concepts in the classification, diagnosis, and management of orbital vascular malformations.

Nomenclature

As our understanding of the histology and flow characteristics for vascular lesions has increased over time, so has our ability to classify them in a rational manner. Moving away from an array of disjointed naming systems focused on specific lesions such as hemangioma, lymphangioma, varix, etc., modern classification systems unify terminology as it relates to pathophysiologic characteristics.

The earliest classification systems were based on endothelial cell type [1], and later refined to include characteristics of intralesional flow [2, 3], resulting in a comprehensive systemic classification system now espoused by the International Society for the Study of Vascular Anomalies (ISSVA) [4]. This system allows for rational treatment and consistent scientific discussion (Table 2.1).

S. Ramesh · D. Rootman (✉)
Department of Orbital and Ophthalmic Plastic Surgery, UCLA Stein Eye Institute,
Los Angeles, CA, USA
e-mail: Ramesh@jsei.ucla.edu; Rootman@jsei.ucla.edu

© Springer Nature Singapore Pte Ltd. 2019
A. Gupta, P. Tahiliani (eds.), *Orbit and Oculoplastics*, Current Practices in
Ophthalmology, https://doi.org/10.1007/978-981-13-8538-4_2

Table 2.1 ISSVA 2014 Classification of vascular anomalies

Tumors		Malformations	
Infantile hemangioma		Fast	Slow
Tufted angioma	Arterial	Arteriovenous malformation Fistula	Capillary Port wine mark Telangectasia
Kaposiform hemangioendothelioma	Venous		Distensible Non-distensible Cavernous malformation
Hemangiopericytoma	Lymphatic		Macrocystic: deep Microcystic: superficial
Pyogenic granuloma Spindle cell hemangioendothelioma	Mixed	Capillary-venous	Venolymphatic Venous dominant Lymphatic dominant

The ISSVA classification at its base level separates vascular tumors from malformations (Table 2.1). Vascular tumors are benign or malignant endothelial neoplasms which grow by abnormal cell proliferation. These are rarely present at birth and grow out of phase with the patient. Most commonly represented tumors of this group are infantile hemangioma, hemangiopericytoma, and hemangioendothelioma. These lesions are beyond the scope of the present discussion, which will focus solely on vascular malformations.

Vascular malformations are congenital lesions likely related to an embryologic error in the development. They tend to grow proportionally with the patient and are present throughout the life. Vascular malformations are subdivided based on vessel type (arterial, venous, lymphatic, or mixed) and flow characteristics (fast or slow).

Mixed lesions involve arterial, venous, and/or lymphatic components and represent a spectrum of disease. The most common of these phenotypes is the combined venolymphatic malformation, formerly known as lymphangioma.

Morphologic considerations within lesion type and flow categories further characterize malformations in important ways for diagnosis and management, particularly in the orbit [5]. Venous components are divided into distensible and non-distensible subtypes, lymphatic into microcystic and macrocystic morphologic groups, and venolymphatic malformations further characterized as lymphatic- or venous-dominant.

Imaging

Imaging modalities can be described as noninvasive (ultrasound, computed tomography (CT), and magnetic resonance imaging (MRI)) or invasive (catheter angiography), and further characterized as static or dynamic. Static imaging traditionally provides information regarding soft tissue components. Bony features on static imaging may be better assessed with computed tomography (CT), which is also useful for the identification of phleboliths, providing some clues regarding flow characteristics. Static magnetic resonance imaging (MRI) protocols provide better soft tissue differentiation, with generally higher resolution. Additionally, information regarding tissue composition characteristics can be derived through comparison of relative signal intensity on T1 and T2 weighted sequences. Fat suppression is highly valuable in differentiating normal from abnormal orbital tissues that may both be relatively bright on T1 and T2 imaging.

Dynamic, time-resolved imaging is indispensable in evaluating vascular disease. Catheter angiography is likely the gold standard for such imaging, and may be combined with intravascular interventions to treat lesions in many circumstances. However, such interventions do carry some risk and it is ideal to evaluate with non-invasive imaging in advance of interventional procedures. These investigations are helpful in deciding whether angiography is appropriate and in planning for possible intravascular interventions with or without concurrent or subsequent surgery.

Dual-phase CT angiography (CTA) with post-contrast imaging in both arterial and venous phases can be useful in evaluating the progression of intralesional filling characteristics. The addition of Valsalva maneuver during the venous phase can be invaluable in the identification of distensible components that may not be identified clinically [6] and in the assessment of post Valsalva spatial relationships. Time resolved MRI sequences (TRICKS sequence, GE Healthcare, Wauwatosa, WI or TWIST sequence, Siemens Corporation, Washington DC, among others) can provide information regarding the phase of filling for different aspects of the lesions. They are however limited in spatial resolution and do not reveal washout or drainage patterns well due to luminal wall staining.

These various dynamic imaging modalities can provide invaluable information regarding composition (arterial or venous, based on time resolution), flow (distensibility and flow voids), and anatomic relationships (inflow and outflow pathways) that may be critical to optimal management. Specific imaging applications will be discussed in the appropriate sections below.

Arterial

Arteriovenous Fistula (AVF)

Pathophysiology
AVFs are rare lesions composed of a single, direct connection between the arterial and venous systems. These are not true embryologic malformations, but rather acquired lesions that may be spontaneous or initiated by trauma [7].

Clinical Features
Orbital AVFs present with typical congestive signs including proptosis (potentially pulsatile), chemosis, tortuous episcleral vasculature, and elevated intraocular pressure. Cavernous sinus findings may be evident, if the fistula is intra-cavernous, and may include motor and/or sensory nerve dysfunction. Intra-orbital fistula can occur

and may not demonstrate these classic findings [8]. Fundus examination may show venous engorgement and/or tortuosity. Proptosis is typically not enhanced with Valsalva or positioning, although venous engorgement may be exacerbated.

Imaging

Static imaging may reveal a dilated superior ophthalmic vein (SOV) along with orbital congestion and engorgement of the extraocular muscles. Cavernous sinus expansion may also be noted. Contrast enhanced imaging may further delineate the increased orbital vascularity, however, is not particularly additive to other static imaging. Non-invasive angiography (CTA or MR angiography (MRA)) may be able to demonstrate fistulous changes, although catheter angiography is often required for both diagnosis and management.

Treatment

Treatment often involves endovascular embolization or coiling. The fistula is typically approached endovascularly via a transfemoral venous or arterial access point. Rarely, direct cannulation of the SOV or other approaches utilizing lesser vessels of the face are required for access. Angiography may reveal a foreign body in case of traumatic etiology, and removal of the foreign body may be sufficient to allow closure of the fistula [7].

Arteriovenous Malformations (AVM)

Pathophysiology

AVMs are rare fast-flow lesions composed of tangles of arterial vessels which anastomose directly with veins, bypassing a capillary bed (Fig. 2.1). Histology demonstrates thick-walled musculature often with intrastromal hemorrhage, deficiencies in elastic layers and a nidus of cellular stroma between vessels [9]. This stroma may have a role in secreting cytokines that propagate the lesion [9]. They typically occur in anastomotic zones, and may be associated with retinal or cerebral AVMs, both syndromic (e.g., Wyburn-Mason) or non-syndromic in nature.

Clinical Features

Orbital AVMs typically present with mass effect, swelling, proptosis with or without ocular pulsations, bruit, and/or pain. Valsalva maneuver may unmask pulsatile proptosis. Rarely, vision loss from a steal syndrome, intralesional thrombosis, or hemorrhage can be the presenting symptom. Stimuli for growth include pregnancy, menarche and trauma, and lesions may be diagnosed around these times [9].

Imaging

Noncontrast imaging may only show a poorly-defined soft tissue mass with or without flow voids (Fig. 2.1b, d). Early phase CT or MR angiography may demonstrate

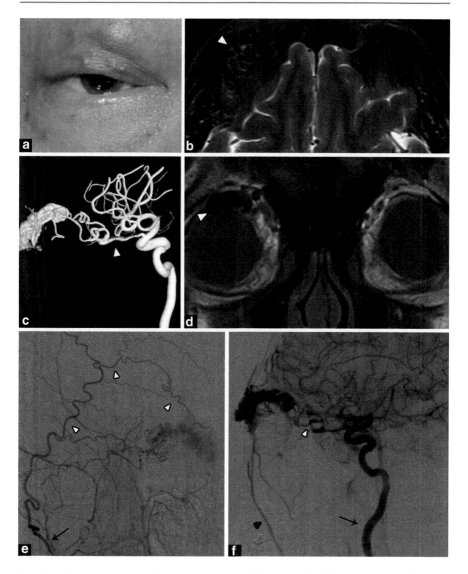

Fig. 2.1 Patient with right orbital arteriovenous malformation (AVM). Clinical photo (**a**) shows bluish subcutaneous discoloration and ptosis due to mass effect in the upper eyelid. Axial T2-weighted MRI with fat suppression (**b**) and coronal T1-weighted MRI with fat suppression and contrast enhancement (**d**) showing orbital AVM in the right superior orbit with dilated, tortuous vessels and flow voids (arrowhead). MR angiogram with 3D reconstruction (**c**) shows the lesion in detail with the primary feeding artery (ophthalmic artery, arrowhead) arising from the internal carotid artery. Catheter angiography from the external carotid (**e**, arrow) shows a secondary feeder from the superficial temporal artery (arrowheads) with slow filling of the lesion. Catheter angiography from the internal carotid (**f**, arrow) reveals brisk filling of the lesion through the ophthalmic artery (white arrowhead) and drainage through the facial vein (black arrowhead)

distinct vessels, although late phase sequences may simply show diffuse enhancement in the mass. Time-resolved MRI reveals arterial-phase filling within a distinct tangle of vessels. The venous phase of MRI sequences is poorly defined due to the collection of contrast in the vessels. Doppler ultrasound can demonstrate fast flow characteristics.

Invasive angiography is the standard for diagnosis and characteristically demonstrates early arterial flow of contrast into the distinct vessels, often followed by a blush of contrast into the smaller abnormal arterioles. Inflow is often derived from multiple feeder branches of both the internal and external carotid (Fig. 2.1e, f). Outflow is via significantly dilated and engorged veins leading variably to the facial veins, cavernous sinus, pterygoid plexus and/or anomalous communicating veins to the intracranial sinuses.

Treatment

Observation typically follows growth over time, periodically interrupted by thrombosis or hemorrhage events. Direct excision can be attempted; however, poorly defined borders make the lesion difficult to completely excise, and large inflow channels can lead to significant intraoperative bleeding. Intravascular embolization alone can be performed, however, recurrence is common. Management of arterial inflow with intravascular embolization and complete excision may be the best option for management. Complete excision offers the greatest chance for limiting recurrence, although this should be balanced with the functional and/or cosmetic consequences of such a procedure. Adjunctive sclerotherapy, laser and/or embolization may be useful in cases where incomplete resection may be necessary to preserve essential function and cosmesis.

Venous

Cavernous Venous Malformation

Pathophysiology

Cavernous venous malformations, previously known as cavernous hemangiomas, are common lesions (up to 9% of orbital masses [10]) that typically present in middle age, more commonly among females [11] (Fig. 2.2). The hemangioma label is likely inaccurate as they do not represent abnormally proliferating cells, but rather a collection of low-flow blood vessels growing slowly by the normal vascular processes of thrombosis and recanalization [12].

Cavernous malformations typically have a robust external capsule which may incorporate adjacent neurovasculature (e.g., the ophthalmic artery) as the lesion grows, particularly in the orbital apex [13]. Histologically, lesions are composed of dilated vascular channels with areas of thrombosis in a fibrous stroma. They can have a lobular structure and intralesional fat [13]. Endothelial cells express vascular endothelial growth factor (VEGF) and contain extensive smooth muscle actin (SMA)-positive myofibroblasts [12].

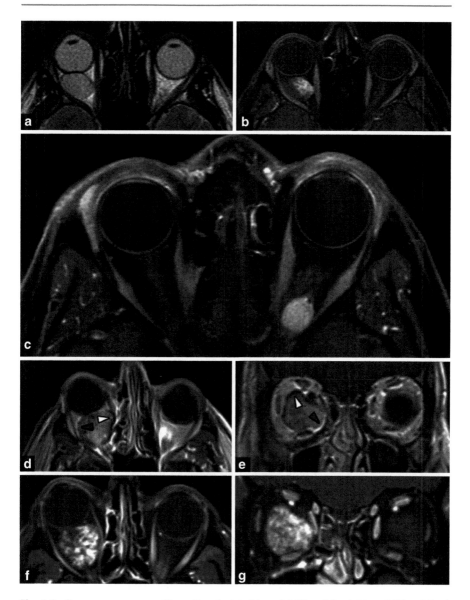

Fig. 2.2 Cavernous venous malformation depicted in axial T2-weighted (**a**) and T1-weighted post-contrast MRI (**b**) with the typical, intraconal location, indentation of the posterior aspect of the globe, and early, high-intensity enhancement. A posterior cavernous venous malformation with extension through the superior orbital fissure to the cavernous sinus shown in axial T1-weighted contrast-enhanced MRI (**c**); the anterior components of this lesion were exsanguinated and debulked transorbitally, allowing for sufficient reduction in proptosis to relieve the patient's optic neuropathy and uncontrolled pain. Cavernous venous malformation depicted in axial and coronal T2-weighted MRI (**d**, **e**) showing an intraconal location and the "double artifact sign" with a black line on the outer edge of the lesion (white arrowhead) and white line on the inner edge of the opposite edge of the lesion (black arrowhead). Contrast-enhanced T1-weighted image with fat suppression (**f**, **g**) of the same patient shows early, high-intensity enhancement

Clinical Features

Many lesions are discovered incidentally on brain imaging, and as such are asymptomatic. However, up to one third of patients do describe vague symptoms of dull orbital pain and/or headache, leading to brain imaging and lesion discovery [12]. Most often they present with slowly worsening proptosis [14]. Motility restriction, gaze-evoked amaurosis, diplopia and optic neuropathy are less common symptoms. Differential diagnosis includes hemangiopericytoma/solitary fibrous tumor, schwannoma, infantile hemangioma, and venolymphatic malformation.

Imaging

Static imaging demonstrates a well-defined, typically intraconal lesion, often in the middle third of the orbit [12]. These tend to indent rather than mold to the globe, are smooth bordered, spherical, and of variable internal density. Apical lesions may have intracranial extension through the superior orbital fissure (Fig. 2.2c).

On MRI, lesions are isointense to gray matter on T1 and hyperintense on T2, and may exhibit the "double artifact sign," which is a black line on the inner edge of the lesion and a white line on the outer edge of the opposite side of the lesion (Fig. 2.2d, e). Static contrast enhanced studies demonstrate late uniform enhancement (Fig. 2.2a, b) [15]. Due to the long capture time with MRI, differences in contrast enhancement may be noted from one sequence to the next. Examination of earlier sequences after contrast injection show high intensity multifocal enhancement, while images acquired later show diffuse, moderate enhancement (Fig. 2.2f, g). Dual phase CTA delineates the slow inflow characteristics of these lesions with patchy focal or multifocal enhancement early and diffuse moderate enhancement later [16].

Treatment

Lesions can be observed if symptoms are limited and tolerable. Treatment typically consists of surgical excision, where the lesion can be excised with the capsule intact. Exsanguination can assist with removal by reducing the size of the lesion. Care should be taken to ensure the lesion is not fixed to adjacent neurovasculature, especially in the apex.

Complex or apical lesions may also be treated with fractionated stereotactic radiotherapy (40 Gy in 20 sessions), and although this treatment does not typically lead to a large reduction in lesion size, it can be very effective in treating optic neuropathy [17]. Of note, posterior/apical lesions extending into the superior orbital fissure may resolve with even partial resection, possibly due to secondary induced thrombosis of residual mass [13].

Distensible and Non-distensible Venous Malformations

Pathophysiology

Venous malformations are comprised of distensible (enlarge with Valsalva) and/or non-distensible components. These lesions may arise from either a congenital weakness in the wall of a post-capillary venule (i.e., varix) or from dysmorphic vein formation [16]. Internally, lesions can exhibit spongy, cavitary or dysmorphic morphology [18]. Outflow can be isolated into normal veins and ectatic veins, or the lesion as a whole can be completely ectatic [18]. Outflow anatomy is varied and can drain through single or multiple tributary networks into the cavernous sinus, pterygopalatine fossa, facial vasculature, and/or intracranial sinuses. Lesions may be isolated, in a combined venolymphatic malformation or as part of systemic vascular dysmorphism syndromes.

Clinical Features

Venous malformations are congenital lesions that typically present in the second or third decade of life without a predilection for either sex. Symptoms may include pressure sensation or pain and wasting and/or enophthalmos due to orbital fat atrophy after repeated episodes of hemorrhage and/or proptosis [19]. Distensible lesions are often associated with Valsalva-induced symptomatology including pain, vision loss and diplopia under conditions of elevated venous pressure such as bending and straining. Signs may also be Valsalva-induced and can include induction of an afferent pupillary defect, motility restriction and/or proptosis. Hemorrhage or thrombosis can occur and in these situations pateints may note sudden onset of pain and vision loss with or without ecchymosis in these situations. It is noteworthy that clinical changes with Valsalva may be evident in only 60% of patients with a radiologically dynamic lesion [6]. Non-distensible lesions may present with spontaneous hemorrhage due to the inability of the vessel to respond to changes in flow [18].

Speed of onset and subsequent resolution of distension on Valsalva maneuver provides clues as to the inflow and outflow characteristics of the lesion. Slow-filling or emptying lesions may have small and/or multifocal inflow or outflow networks, respectively, while faster-filling or emptying lesions will typically be associated with larger and more ectatic connections with the venous system.

Imaging

Static imaging may show a poorly defined soft tissue mass with variable enhancement with or without phleboliths. Non-distensible components may demonstrate early pooling of contrast. However, smaller or extremely collapsible lesions may be difficult to identify at all on static imaging (Fig. 2.3). Dynamic imaging is invaluable in assessing these lesions, and significant components of the lesion may be revealed (Fig. 2.3) with a Valsalva maneuver performed approximately 1 min after contrast administration. Large venous channels with complex inflow and outflow as well as small arterial components may also be identified (Figs. 2.4 and 2.5) [20].

Treatment

Indications for intervention include persistent pain, a functional deficit such as globe dystopia, vision loss, strabismus or cosmesis. Smaller, very low-flow lesions in the anterior orbit may be excised completely with meticulous surgical technique and standard hemostatic maneuvers. However, it is often prudent to manage these lesions in conjunction with invasive angiography teams.

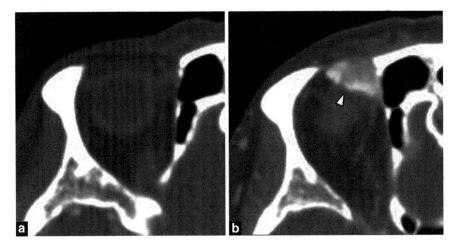

Fig. 2.3 Axial CT of orbital venous malformation with contrast, pre-Valsalva (**a**) and post-Valsalva (**b**) maneuver, highlighting the distensible nature of the lesion (arrowhead)

Direct puncture is the most focused access technique, and this can be performed after exposing the lesion surgically or in a percutaneous manner. Intraoperative Valsalva can be useful in expanding the target for puncture and can be induced by elevating the intrathoracic pressure with the help of the anesthesiologist. Puncture can be followed by mapping, and outflow channels can be assessed for size and drainage pattern.

The goal of this procedure is to control the lesion while avoiding collateral damage to the downstream structures. This can be accomplished in many ways. Slow-flow lesions with limited and/or safe drainage zones can be sclerosed, often with small aliquots to allow for concentration of agent within the lesion of interest (and dilution downstream). Very slow-flow lesions can be embolized directly with glue starting at the outflow and backfilling into the inflow. Faster-flow lesions may be filled with multiple glue polymerization configurations, with faster polymerizing glue at the outflow regions and more slowly polymerizing glue subsequently. Very fast-outflow channels can be controlled downstream with invasive venography and balloon catheterization, effectively blocking the downstream elements. This can be followed by direct puncture and embolization. Surgical excision of the malformation and embolic material follows in most cases.

Common sclerosants include sodium morrhuate 5%, sodium tetradecyl sulfate 3% (SDS), absolute alcohol, OK-432, bleomycin or tetracyclines [19, 21, 22]. OK-432 induces cytokine release which recruits inflammatory cells and incites thrombus, while the other sclerosants cause direct intimal injury leading to inflammation and thrombosis. Common complications include edema, blistering, or ulceration. Rare but serious complications include cerebral embolism in the presence of a patent foramen ovale, orbital compartment syndrome, or transient neuropathy of adjacent nerves (e.g., CN VII near the masseter) [23, 24]. Care must be taken to limit the amount of sclerosant given (e.g., a maximum of 3–4 mL of SDS foam into the orbit) to avoid complications.

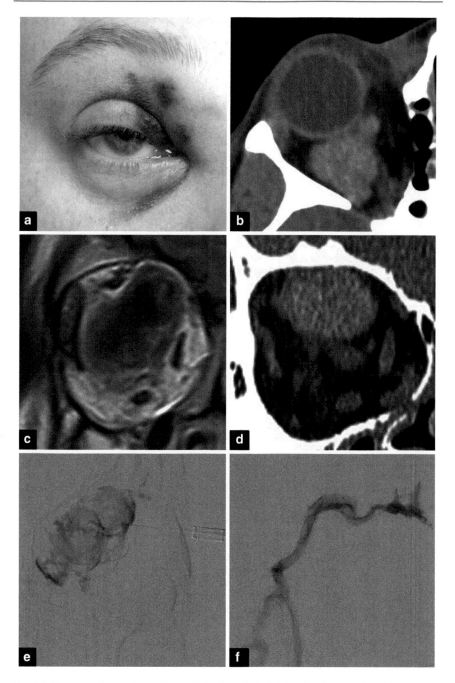

Fig. 2.4 Venous malformation of the orbit. Clinical photo (**a**) showing thrombosis and hemorrhage resulting in acute proptosis and pain, which was improved with oral corticosteroid. Axial and coronal non-contrast CT (**b, d**) showing an irregular soft tissue mass in the intraconal and superior orbit. Coronal T1-weighted MRI (**c**) showing irregular thrombosis within the lesion. Angiography through direct puncture showing slow filling of the lesion (**e**) and outflow through the cavernous sinus (**f**)

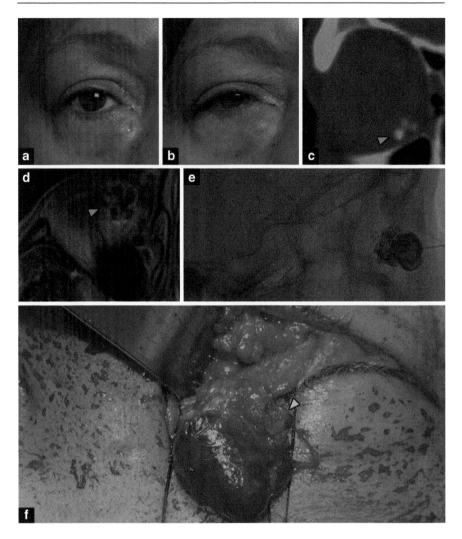

Fig. 2.5 Venous malformation in the inferomedial anterior orbit. Clinical photos pre-Valsalva (**a**) and post-Valsalva (**b**) show enlargement of lesion with edema in the lower lid after the maneuver. Coronal non-contrast CT (**c**) demonstrating phleboliths within the lesion (arrowhead). Axial non-contrast T1-weighted MRI (**d**) with flow voids and/or phleboliths (arrowhead), which appear similar on MRI. Catheter angiography via direct puncture (**e**) and gluing of the lesion with cyanoacrylate facilitates subsequent surgical excision (**f**); cyanoacrylate glue in a cut portion of the lesion is noted (arrowhead)

Common embolizing agents include cyanoacrylate glue (nBCA) and ethylene alcohol vinyl copolymer (Onyx, Medtronic, Northridge, CA). Embolization aids in surgical excision by allowing hemostasis as well as giving the lesion a firmness which allows easier dissection and excision (Fig. 2.5e, f).

Lymphatic/Combined

Venolymphatic Malformations

Pathophysiology

It is now generally recognized that the entity formerly known as lymphangioma, is more accurately described as a venolymphatic malformation. This is due to the persistence of both venous and lymphatic elements in the lesions and a lack of abnormally proliferating clonal cells more typical of lesions designated by "-oma." These lesions exist on a physiologic spectrum from venous-dominant to lymphatic-dominant, with some suggesting there are few if any truly isolated lymphatic lesions [25]. Morphologically, these malformations may be comprised of macrocystic (large, individually identifiable cysts) and microcystic (smaller, less distinct cysts) components, again existing on a spectrum of varying proportions of each.

Theories of their genesis generally suggest that they may be formed from arborization or embryonic sequestration of venous structures. The orbit is generally devoid of lymphatics and lymphatic and venous vessels share an embryologic predecessor [26]. Other theories presume that blood-derived cells may differentiate into lymphatic elements.

Vessels in the lymphatic components generally do not contain significant numbers of erythrocytes (unless a recent hemorrhage is evident), and flow is nonexistent or very slow. Lesions are mostly not encapsulated and tend not to respect tissue boundaries or anatomic planes, often interdigitating with and through adjacent structures. Some primarily macrocystic lesions can be somewhat encapsulated and certain lesions may demonstrate an internal and external lobular architecture (Fig. 2.7).

Clinical Features

Lymphatic malformations are relatively common congenital orbital lesions and may remain clinically unapparent until the early teens. They typically grow slowly although can be punctuated by episodes of hemorrhage characterized by acute onset of pain, proptosis, and vision loss due to rapid expansion of cystic elements ("chocolate cysts"). They may also expand at the time of antecedent respiratory tract infection leading to proliferation of the stromal immune system elements (e.g., follicles). Presenting signs include proptosis (with or without optic neuropathy), strabismus and ptosis. Blood-filled or xanthochromic cysts may be observed in the conjunctiva with bluish subcutaneous cysts in the eyelid. Venous elements may present in a similar fashion as described in previous sections regarding venous malformations.

Imaging

Static imaging may reveal macrocysts with or without fluid–fluid levels. These are often best identified on T2-weighted MRI sequences (Fig. 2.6b, c). Microcystic regions appear as poorly defined, diffusely enhancing and infiltrative masses (Fig. 2.6d). Dynamic imaging may demonstrate inflow character and/or internal

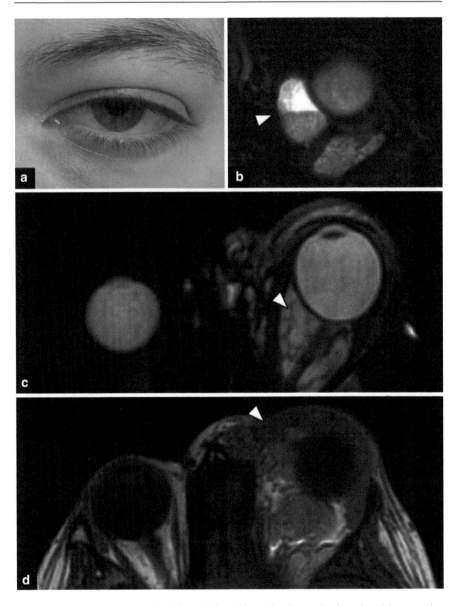

Fig. 2.6 Clinical photo of an orbital lymphatic malformation in a pediatric patient (**a**), presenting with chemosis, edema and fullness after an antecedent upper respiratory tract infection. Axial T2-weighted contrast-enhanced MRI (**b**) shows a large macrocyst with a fluid–fluid level. Axial T2-weighted post-contrast and T1-weighted non-contrast MRI of another pediatric patient with orbital lymphatic dominant malformation (**c, d**) depicting intraconal macrocysts (**c**, arrowhead) with an anterior microcystic component in the eyelid (**d**, arrowhead)

vascular architecture. Flow voids and/or phleboliths may be evident. Venous components are best defined on Valsalva-augmented sequences. Differential diagnosis includes cavernous venous malformations, infantile hemangioma, and orbital inflammatory disease.

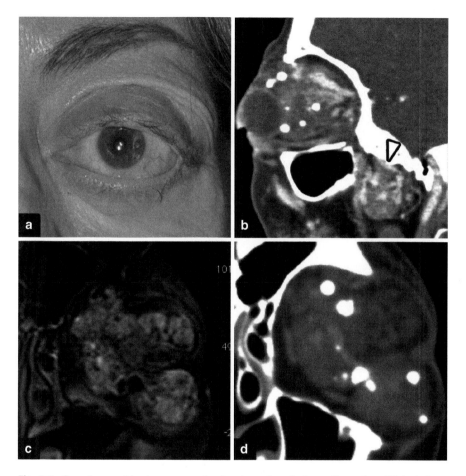

Fig. 2.7 Complex combined venous-predominant venolymphatic malformation. Clinical photo (**a**) demonstrates proptosis. Contrast-enhanced CT (**b, d, f**) and T1-weighted MRI (**c, e**) demonstrate a complex lesion with intraconal, extraconal and eyelid involvement, numerous phleboliths, and infiltration of orbital soft tissues as well as the pterygopalatine fossa (**b**, arrowhead). Catheter angiography via direct puncture (**g**) shows the internal architecture of a lobular lymphatic component, and another superolateral microcystic lymphatic component with minimal connection to the medial portion. Immunohistochemistry shows rich staining for vascular endothelial growth factor (VEGF) (**h**, brown)

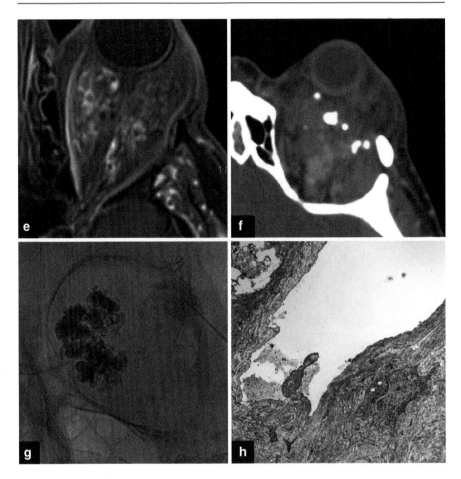

Fig. 2.7 (continued)

Treatment

Lesions may be observed for many years as asymptomatic; while they are unlikely to regress, they may stop growing at adulthood [25]. The infiltrative nature of such lesions makes them poorly amenable in most cases to complete surgical excision due to the involvement of vital orbital structures. Incomplete management is often followed by recurrent growth. Sclerosing therapy has become the mainstay of management and may involve the use of various agents including sodium morrhuate, sodium tetradecyl sulfate, OK-432, or bleomycin. This can be performed with direct puncture in an outpatient or surgical setting for smaller, anteriorly located lesions or under fluoroscopic guidance in conjunction with interventional radiology. The latter technique has the advantage of understanding complex interactions between these lesions and internal venous components and can assure adequate treatment breadth. Recent advances in our understanding of the biochemistry in these lesions suggest a role for VEGF mediated processes in the development and propagation of venolymphatic malformations [25]. In the future, VEGF blocking agents may be useful in the management of these malformations (Fig. 2.7g). Whatever the methodology, lesions may require multiple treatments for adequate management.

Summary

Thorough understanding of the flow characteristics and anatomic distribution of a vascular malformation is critical to optimal treatment. Advances in biomaterials, fluoroscopy-guided therapy, and our understanding of the pathophysiology of these lesions have contributed to better management. Future research should strive to understand the embryologic and biochemical pathways by which these lesions grow, to provide a targeted therapy with powerful and durable effect.

Pearls and Pitfalls

- Pearl #1: Understanding the flow characteristics of each lesion is key to optimal treatment.
- Pearl #2: A multidisciplinary approach with interventional radiology aids in addressing complex lesions.
- Pitfall #1: Improper nomenclature confuses understanding and inhibits optimal treatment.
- Pitfall #2: Primary surgical excision has a high risk of hemorrhage, collateral damage, or incomplete excision with recurrence of.

References

1. Mulliken JB, Glowacki J. Hemangiomas and vascular malformations in infants and children: a classification based on endothelial characteristics. Plast Reconstr Surg. 1982;69:412–22.
2. Garzon MC, Huang JT, Enjolras O, Frieden IJ. Vascular malformations: part i. J Am Acad Dermatol. 2007;56:353–70. quiz 71-4.
3. Jackson IT, Carreno R, Potparic Z, Hussain K. Hemangiomas, vascular malformations, and lymphovenous malformations: classification and methods of treatment. Plast Reconstr Surg. 1993;91:1216–30.
4. Issva classification of vascular anomalies. ISSVA General Assembly, Melbourne, Australia; 2014. issva.org/classification.
5. Harris GJ. Orbital vascular malformations: a consensus statement on terminology and its clinical implications. Orbital society. Am J Ophthalmol. 1999;127(4):453–5.
6. Rootman J, Heran MK, Graeb DA. Vascular malformations of the orbit: classification and the role of imaging in diagnosis and treatment strategies∗. Ophthal Plast Reconstr Surg. 2014;30:91–104.
7. Yazc B, Yazc Z, Erdogan C, Rootman J. Intraorbital arteriovenous fistula secondary to penetrating injury. Ophthalmic Plast Reconstr Surg. 2007;23:275–8.
8. Konstas AA, Rootman DB, Quiros PA, Ross IB. Transarterial embolization of a spontaneous intraorbital arteriovenous fistula with n-bca glue. Ophthalmic Plast Reconstr Surg. 2017;33(3):e63–4.
9. Warrier S, Prabhakaran VC, Valenzuela A, et al. Orbital arteriovenous malformations. Arch Ophthalmol. 2008;126:1669–75.

10. Bonavolonta G, Strianese D, Grassi P, Comune C, et al. An analysis of 2,480 space-occupying lesions of the orbit from 1976 to 2011. Ophthalmic Plast Reconstr Surg. 2013;29(2):79–86.
11. Alfred PRCD. Cavernous hemangiomas of the orbit. Orbit. 1996;15:59–66.
12. Rootman DB, Heran MK, Rootman J, et al. Cavernous venous malformations of the orbit (so-called cavernous haemangioma): a comprehensive evaluation of their clinical, imaging and histologic nature. Br J Ophthalmol. 2014;98:880–8.
13. Harris GJ. Cavernous hemangioma of the orbital apex: Pathogenetic considerations in surgical management. Am J Ophthalmol. 2010;150:764–73.
14. Rootman DB, Rootman J, White VA. Comparative histology of orbital, hepatic and subcutaneous cavernous venous malformations. Br J Ophthalmol. 2015;99:138–40.
15. Khan SN, Sepahdari AR. Orbital masses: CT and MRI of common vascular lesions, benign tumors, and malignancies. Saudi J Ophthalmol. 2012;26:373–83.
16. Heran MK, Rootman J, Sangha BS, Yeo JM. Dynamic arterial and valsalva-augmented venous phase multidetector ct for orbital vascular lesions: a pictorial review∗. Ophthal Plast Reconstr Surg. 2014;30:180–5.
17. Rootman DB, Rootman J, Gregory S, et al. Stereotactic fractionated radiotherapy for cavernous venous malformations (hemangioma) of the orbit. Ophthal Plast Reconstr Surg. 2012;28:96–102.
18. Legiehn GM, Heran MK. Venous malformations: classification, development, diagnosis, and interventional radiologic management. Radiol Clin N Am. 2008;46:545–97, vi.
19. Lacey B, Rootman J, Marotta TR. Distensible venous malformations of the orbit. Ophthalmology. 1999;106:1197–209.
20. Callahan AB, Meyers PM, Garrity JA, et al. Low-flow arterialized venous malformations of the orbit. Ophthal Plast Reconstr Surg. 2017;33:256–60.
21. Schwarcz RM, Ben Simon GJ, Cook T, Goldberg RA. Sclerosing therapy as first line treatment for low flow vascular lesions of the orbit. Am J Ophthalmol. 2006;141:333–9.
22. Stacey AW, Gemmete JJ, Kahana A. Management of orbital and periocular vascular anomalies. Ophthal Plast Reconstr Surg. 2015;31:427–36.
23. Colletti G, Deganello A, Bardazzi A, et al. Complications after treatment of head and neck venous malformations with sodium tetradecyl sulfate foam. J Craniofac Surg. 2017;28:e388–e92.
24. Tessari L, Cavezzi A, Frullini A. Preliminary experience with a new sclerosing foam in the treatment of varicose veins. Dermatol Surg. 2001;27:58–60.
25. Nassiri N, Rootman J, Rootman DB, Goldberg RA. Orbital lymphaticovenous malformations: current and future treatments. Surv Ophthalmol. 2015;60:383–405.
26. Rootman J. Vascular malformations of the orbit: hemodynamic concepts. Orbit. 2009;22:103–20.

Surgical Management of Thyroid Eye Disease: Recent Updates

3

Adit Gupta

Introduction

Thyroid eye disease (TED) is an immunological disorder commonly associated with Grave's disease (GD). Even after years of research, the aetiology remains a mystery due to multiple immune pathways involved [1]. It has profound impact on the patient due to the associated visual, aesthetic and psychosocial sequelae.

Although, it is most commonly associated with GD, it can also be associated with hypothyroidism and a euthyroid status. There is a female predilection (2:1) and a strong association with smoking [2].

Various classification systems have been devised to guide treatment strategies, but there is no foolproof method of grading the disease due to its varied presentation spectrum. This makes the management of TED a dilemma world over.

The treatment strategy for TED is multi-pronged and consists of different modalities such as medical therapy, functional and cosmetic surgery and radiotherapy. Medical therapy ranges from supportive ocular surface protection and lubrication to potent immunosuppressive agents [3]. Recent advances in the form of molecular mediators offer promise to modify the disease in the initial stages avoiding the fibrotic sequelae of TED [4, 5]. Until robust data is obtained about the efficacy of molecular mediators, surgery remains an important tool to manage these unfortunate patients with mechanical and fibrotic sequelae of TED.

In this chapter, we discuss the technological and conceptual advances of minimally invasive keyhole surgeries for TED that offer predictable results with better aesthetics.

A. Gupta (✉)
Mumbai Eye Plastic Surgery Centre, Mumbai, Maharashtra, India

Department of Ophthalmology, Deenanath Mangeshkar Hospital, Pune, Maharashtra, India

Department of Orbital and Ophthalmic Plastic Surgery, UCLA Stein Eye Institute, Los Angeles, CA, USA

© Springer Nature Singapore Pte Ltd. 2019
A. Gupta, P. Tahiliani (eds.), *Orbit and Oculoplastics*, Current Practices in Ophthalmology, https://doi.org/10.1007/978-981-13-8538-4_3

Pathology

The pathophysiology of TED is characterized by the involvement of orbital tissues, such as the orbital fat and extraocular muscles (EOM). There is orbital fibroblast proliferation with deposition of glycosaminoglycans and hyaluronate derivatives leading to an increase in intraorbital pressure and contents, derangement of the ocular surface, eyelid signs or in severe cases, a dysfunction of the optic nerve [6]. This leads to proptosis, eyelid retraction, eyelid lag, ocular surface disorders, diplopia, strabismus and, in extreme cases, visual compromise.

Timing of Surgery?

Surgical rehabilitation in TED is most often carried out in the 'burnt out' phase of the disease when all the inflammation has subsided. We follow a practice of observing the patient for 3–6 months for a stable disease before surgery. Cosmetic indications include correction of the asymmetric proptosis, eyelid retraction and periocular puffiness. Apart from cosmetic indications, surgery is also advised for correction of strabismus and EOM imbalance, correction of disfiguring proptosis leading to ocular surface compromise. Emergency surgical intervention is needed in cases of dysthyroid optic neuropathy to relieve the compression on the optic nerve and to prevent loss of vision.

Components of Rehabilitation

The four components of surgical intervention for TED, if required, in the order of surgery are [7]:

1. Orbital decompression surgery for proptosis
2. Strabismus surgery for extraocular muscle imbalance
3. Eyelid surgery for retraction
4. Aesthetic surgery for soft tissue redraping

Proptosis is usually the most disfiguring complication of TED (Fig. 3.1). It may be unilateral or bilateral and asymmetric. The correction of proptosis usually needs an increase in the orbital cavity space either by drilling the bone or by the removal of orbital fat to reduce the soft tissue volume in the orbit. The number of orbital walls or the amount of orbital fat to be removed depends on the amount of correction needed. The second stage involves correction of the EOM imbalance. In TED, the commonest muscle involved is the inferior rectus causing hypotropia due to tightness. Due to fibrotic changes in the levator muscle, eyelid retraction is another common sign of TED. This is corrected after the strabismus has been corrected. This involves surgeries on the levator aponeurosis which involves either lengthening or recessing it. The final

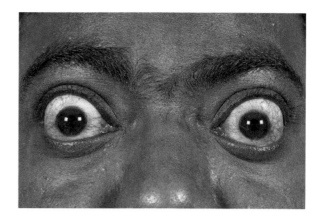

Fig. 3.1 Disfiguring bilateral proptosis in a young male with thyroid eye disease

stage is soft tissue redraping to achieve smooth periorbital contours to negate the periorbital soft tissue hypertrophy that may happen in TED [7].

Imaging

Imaging of the orbit and the surrounding paranasal sinuses (PNS) is very important in the preoperative planning and surgical decision-making for orbital decompression. Although both computerized tomography (CT) scan or magnetic resonance imaging (MRI) can be advised, we prefer a preoperative CT scan in every case scheduled for orbital decompression. A CT scan gives important information about the bony anatomy and the thickness of the orbital walls. It also gives information about the anatomy of the surrounding PNS. In addition, CT gives a good idea about the position of the fovea ethmoidalis and cribriform plate. Although MRI is better to characterize the soft tissue anatomy, a CT scan reliably delineates between 'fat predominant' versus 'muscle predominant' disease [8, 9].

Surgical Management

Orbital Decompression

As a concept, there has been little change in orbital decompression surgery over the past many years. It still represents a lot of drilling and excision for making space to reposition the orbital contents. Nevertheless, there have been rapid strides in the field of orbital decompression thanks to the new breed of super specialized orbital surgeons.

With the newer techniques, orbital decompression is being carried out via keyhole incisions, leading to faster recovery and lesser morbidity compared to the neurosurgical incisions used in the past. Also, the concepts of bone removal and drilling are well defined owing to a better understanding of the orbital anatomy and the imaging techniques.

Typically, fat is approached first in a case of mild proptosis followed by the lateral, medial and inferior walls in that order. As a rule, each wall provides a 2 mm reduction in proptosis and fat removal would provide approximately 2 mm reduction. There are many variations in the approach and techniques depending on the availability of instruments and the training of the surgeon.

Fat Decompression

For very mild cases of proptosis, intraconal fat removal can be considered as the first wall of orbital decompression. This can be approached via conjunctival hidden incisions in the medial and inferior fornix. Trokel and Kazim have published a large series reflecting the safety and efficacy of intraconal fat removal and more recently reported in the successful treatment of compressive optic neuropathy [10]. Removing 2–5 cc of intraconal fat between the lateral rectus and inferior rectus, and if needed, from the superomedial and inferomedial compartments provides additional proptosis reduction in patients with non-woody, freely flowing fat.

As a rule of thumb, fat decompression alone gives 2 mm reduction in the proptosis. Intraconal fat should be debulked under proper visualization as small bleeders need attention to prevent an orbital haemorrhage which could lead to visual compromise.

Lateral Wall Decompression

Over the last decade, the lateral orbital wall has become the first bony wall to be approached for decompression. Goldberg and colleagues have described three areas in the lateral wall that is the lacrimal keyhole, the basin of the inferior orbit and the sphenoid diploe [11]. Based on a preoperative CT scan, the amount of bone to be drilled or carved is planned. The surgery can be performed through a minimally invasive eyelid crease incision which is very well camouflaged (Fig. 3.2). After this, the lacrimal keyhole is carved to increase the exposure of the deep orbit and to make space for the lacrimal gland. Next, a groove is fashioned in the direction of the superior orbital fissure. Deep drilling of the sphenoid diploe can be performed depending on the amount of correction desired. Above the inferior orbital fissure, there is a thick bone which can be hollowed out to make more space. The basin of the inferior orbital fissure is the bone lying anterior to the fissure. This can be removed to the buccal and maxillary sinus mucosa. Following bone removal, the periorbita is opened all along to help the lacrimal gland prolapse out and settle in the keyhole fossa. Also, the intraconal fat can be accessed for a graded removal. With these techniques, the risks of sinus complications are lesser compared with the other approaches. Also, the risks of new onset diplopia have been shown to be lesser in case of lateral wall decompression [12].

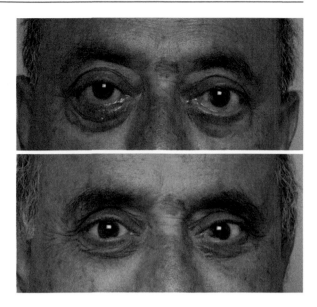

Fig. 3.2 Pre- and post-operative picture of a patient who underwent minimally invasive two-wall decompression and lateral canthal resuspension for thyroid ophthalmopathy. He also had episodes of globe luxation which subsided after the surgery

Medial Wall Decompression

The medial orbital wall has been a favourite with ophthalmologists due to the ease of access. It has become our wall of choice after the lateral wall, for cases where an adequate decompression is not achieved after tackling the lateral wall and fat alone [13]. The medial wall can be approached via a hidden incision in the caruncle or through an endoscopic nasal approach. The medial wall is also the wall of choice for compressive optic neuropathy wherein the posterior medial wall overlying the apex of the orbit and the extraocular muscles can be removed. (Fig. 3.3).

It is important to identify the roof of the ethmoid sinus, the fovea ethmoidalis on preoperative scans to avoid an intraoperative cerebrospinal fluid (CSF) leak.

Inferior Wall/Floor Decompression

The floor of the orbit can be approached by a trans-conjunctival or a subciliary incision. We prefer the trans-conjunctival incision as it can be easily extended laterally to combine it with a lateral wall decompression or medially to tackle the medial wall. Floor decompression usually carries the risk of infraorbital anaesthesia, and so, care must be taken to prevent injury to the infraorbital nerve. It can be combined with a medial wall decompression, especially removal of the posteromedial strut which is removed to achieve deep decompression. The anterior part of the strut should be left avoid hypoglobus.

Complications

Loss of vision: The most dreaded complication of orbital decompression is loss of vision. Visual loss can occur intraoperatively due to vasospasm, ischemia or a direct injury to the optic nerve. It can happen postoperatively due to orbital haemorrhage.

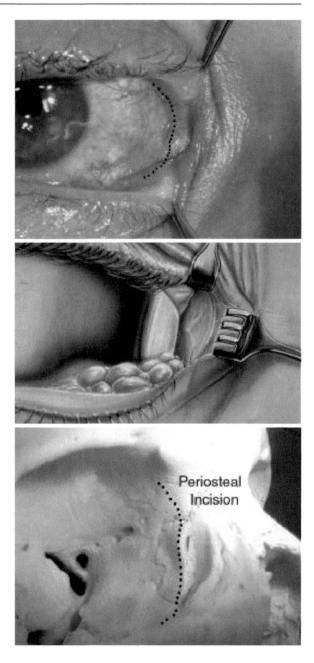

Fig. 3.3 The transcaruncular incision provides wide, rapid access to the entire medial wall for medial and inferomedial decompression. (Regents of the University of California, printed with permission)

The occurrence of vision loss after decompression is extremely rare and can be avoided by gentle surgical technique and proper haemostasis. Also, a close watch for orbital hematoma postoperatively is mandatory in all cases [14].

Cerebrospinal fluid (CSF) leak: CSF leak can occur during a medial decompression from the fovea ethmoidalis or from exposure of the dura in a deep lateral decompression. Most of the leaks are self-limiting. Rarely, a dural repair is needed in cases of persistent leakage [14].

Diplopia: New onset diplopia is the commonest complication that may arise after orbital decompression. It is more common after an unbalanced inferomedial decompression. Usually, it resolves over a period of 3 months. A second stage strabismus surgery may be warranted if the double vision persists beyond 3 months.

Numbness: Numbness of the cheek and the upper lip is a distinct possibility due to an injury to the infraorbital nerve following floor decompression. This usually resolves over a period of 6 months. Permanent numbness might result from a more severe damage to the nerve.

Strabismus Surgery for Extraocular Muscle Imbalance

Restrictive strabismus occurs in 17–51% of patients with TED, whereas diplopia as an initial presentation occurs in 15–20% [15, 16]. Conservative measures, such as the use of prisms for smaller deviations or monocular occlusion are preferred for diplopia during the active phase. Botulinum toxin injection is an option for thyroid myopathy during the active stage of the disease although there is limited data in literature about this [17]. Strabismus surgery is usually carried out after an orbital decompression surgery. Inferior rectus (IR) muscle is the most commonly involved muscle and IR recession is the most commonly performed procedures. Having a realistic expectation from strabismus surgery is important as achieving binocular single vision in all gazes might not be possible in patients where fibrotic changes have set in [18].

Eyelid Surgery for Retraction

Eyelid retraction is one of the commonest eyelid changes seen in a case of TED. Retraction can be seen in the active as well as the chronic phase of the disease. There are various surgical and medical modalities to correct eyelid retraction.

Levator recession surgery can be performed by a trans-cutaneous or a trans-conjunctival approach [19]. The results of surgery are unpredictable, and repeat surgery may be needed in some cases. Recently, a nonsurgical correction using hyaluronic acid gel (HAG) injections is gaining popularity [20]. It is a minimally invasive procedure with lesser recovery time. This can also be performed in the active stage of the disease and is preferable in patients in whom cosmesis is a major concern (Fig. 3.4). The HAG is proposed to mechanically stretch the levator and add weight to the upper eyelid causing lowering of the eyelid position. Eyelid retraction correction also helps reduce surface exposure and dry eye symptoms by reducing the palpebral aperture.

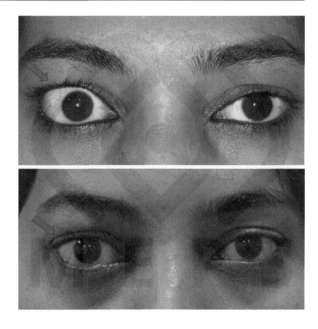

Fig. 3.4 Pre- and post-procedure picture of upper eyelid retraction corrected with 1 cc of hyaluronic acid gel (HAG) injection. Notice the change in upper eyelid position (blue arrows)

Aesthetic Correction

The final stage of TED rehabilitation is an aesthetic correction of the periocular complex. This involves redraping and contouring of the periorbital soft tissues involving a conservative blepharoplasty surgery to remove excessive fat or injections of HAG fillers to fill out the hollows. Botulinum toxin injections are often used to soften hypertrophic glabellar musculature which is frequently observed in TED.

Although surgical management of TED has seen paradigm changes over the past decade, arresting the disease at the molecular level is the future. Recent developments including the use of immunomodulators to treat the disease in its active stage show promise and may be the future. Until then, surgical management helps improve the congestion due to the orbitopathy and improve cosmesis in patients with this disease.

References

1. Naik VM, Naik MN, Goldberg RA, Smith TJ, Douglas RS. Immunopathogenesis of thyroid eye disease: emerging paradigms. Surv Ophthalmol. 2010;55:215–26.
2. Boboridis KG, Bunce C. Surgical orbital decompression for thyroid eye disease. Cochrane Database Syst Rev. 2011;12:CD007630.
3. Bartalena L. Consensus statement of the European group on graves' orbitopathy (EUGOGO) on management of graves' orbitopathy. Thyroid. 2008;18(3):333–46.
4. Salvi M, et al. Small dose of rituximab for graves orbitopathy: new insights into the mechanism of action. Arch Ophthalmol. 2012;130(1):122–4.
5. Briceño CA, Gupta S, Douglas RS. Advances in the management of thyroid eye disease. Int Ophthalmol Clin. 2013;53(3):93–101.

6. Shan SJ, Douglas RS. The pathophysiology of thyroid eye disease. J Neuroophthalmol. 2014;34(2):177–85.
7. Shorr N, Seiff SR. The four stages of surgical rehabilitation of the patient with dysthyroid ophthalmopathy. Ophthalmology. 1986;93:476–83.
8. Gandhi RA, Nair AG. Role of imaging in the management of neuro-ophthalmic disorders. Indian J Ophthalmol. 2011;59:111–6.
9. Naik MN, Nair AG, Gupta A, Kamal S. Minimally invasive surgery for thyroid eye disease. Indian J Ophthalmol. 2015;63(11):847–53.
10. Kazim M, Trokel SL, Acaroglu G, Elliott A. Reversal of dysthyroid optic neuropathy following orbital fat decompression. Br J Ophthalmol. 2000;84:600–5.
11. Goldberg RA, Kim A, Kerivan KM. The lacrimal keyhole, orbital door jamb, and basin of the inferior orbital fissure. Three areas of deep bone in the lateral orbit. Arch Ophthalmol. 2000;116:1618–24.
12. Goldberg RA, Perry JD, Hortaleza V, Tong JT. Strabismus after balanced medial plus lateral wall versus lateral wall only orbital decompression for dysthyroid orbitopathy. Ophthal Plast Reconstr Surg. 2000;16:271–7.
13. Shorr N, Baylis HI, Goldberg RA, Perry JD. Transcaruncular approach to the medial orbit and orbital apex. Ophthalmology. 2000;107:1459–63.
14. Sellari-Franceschini S, Dallan I, Bajraktari A, et al. Surgical complications in orbital decompression for graves' orbitopathy. Acta Otorhinolaryngol Ital. 2016;36(4):265–74.
15. Lee HBH, Rodgers IR, Woog JJ. Evaluation and management of graves' orbitopathy. Otolaryngol Clin N Am. 2006;39:923–42.
16. De Waard R, Koorneef L, Verbatin B Jr. Motility disturbances in graves' ophthalmopathy. Doc Ophthalmol. 1983;56:41–7.
17. Lyons CJ, Vickers SF, Lee JP. Botulinum toxin therapy in dysthyroid strabismus. Eye. 1990;4:538–40.
18. Wallang B, Kekunnaya R, Granet D. Strabismus surgery in thyroid-related eye disease: strategic decision making. Curr Ophthalmol Rep. 2013;1:218–28.
19. Elner VM, Hassan AS, Frueh BR. Graded full-thickness anterior blepharotomy for upper eyelid retraction. Arch Ophthalmol. 2004;122:55–60.
20. Goldberg RA, Lee S, Jayasundera T, Tsirbas A, Douglas RS, McCann JD. Treatment of lower eyelid retraction by expansion of the lower eyelid with hyaluronic acid gel. Ophthal Plast Reconstr Surg. 2007;23:343–8.

Dacryology: Current and Emerging Trends

4

Mohammad Javed Ali

Modern medicine has witnessed evolution and establishment of numerous subspecialties, and dacryology is one such recent addition to the list [1–3]. Dacryology is the science of tears and its drainage through the lacrimal system into the nasal cavity. This branch is mostly practiced by ophthalmologists (mainly the oculoplastic surgeons) and otorhinolaryngologists. The chapter focusses on the advances in this newer subspecialty of dacryology over the past few years.

Introduction

The science of dacryology is progressing at a rapid pace taking leaps and bound in both clinical and basic sciences arena across the globe. There is an increasing interest in this subspecialty of ophthalmic plastic surgery and this augurs well for both the science and the patients it deals with. The advances in recent past are numerous [4, 5] and outside the purview of this chapter. The authors however discuss 12 of them in brief, where they have been directly involved in the past 3 years.

Etiopathogenesis of PANDO: The Gender Angle

Primary acquired nasolacrimal duct obstruction (PANDO) is a clinical syndrome and one of its most recognized feature is the female preponderance. Recent qualitative hormonal analyses have shown the presence of numerous hormonal receptors with variable distribution patterns across the lacrimal drainage system [6]. These include estrogen alpha (ERα), estrogen beta (ERβ), aromatase (CYP19), oxytocin (OXTR), progesterone (PGR), testosterone (TSTR), prolactin (PRL), and

M. J. Ali (✉)
Govindram Seksaria Institute of Dacryology, LV Prasad Eye Institute,
Hyderabad, Telangana, India

© Springer Nature Singapore Pte Ltd. 2019
A. Gupta, P. Tahiliani (eds.), *Orbit and Oculoplastics*, Current Practices in
Ophthalmology, https://doi.org/10.1007/978-981-13-8538-4_4

Fig. 4.1 Immuno-histochemistry microphotograph showing high expression of estrogen alpha receptors in the lacrimal drainage epithelia (ERα, ×200)

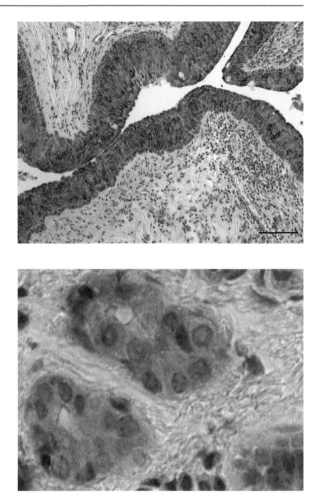

Fig. 4.2 Immuno-histochemistry microphotograph showing prolactin receptor expression in the sub mucosal glands of the lacrimal sac (PRL, ×400)

somatostain receptors 1–5 (Figs. 4.1 and 4.2). Estrogen alpha and beta and aromatase were predominantly epithelial in location, progesterone and testosterone to the basement membranes, stomatostatins to the adluminal vilus surfaces, and oxytocin and prolactin to the cavernous blood vessels and sub mucosal glands, respectively. There were specific patterns and distinctive distribution of receptor expression in healthy males, healthy females and diseased individuals. There is a strong possibility of hormonal micro-environments which are likely to influence the functions and anti-inflammatory milieu in the lacrimal drainage system.

Ultrastructure of Lacrimal System

Recently, ultrastructural anatomy of lacrimal system has been revisited with scanning electron microscopy (SEM; Fig. 4.3). SEM study of normal adult lacrimal system revealed the presence of distinct features of canalicular valves, specific orbicularis

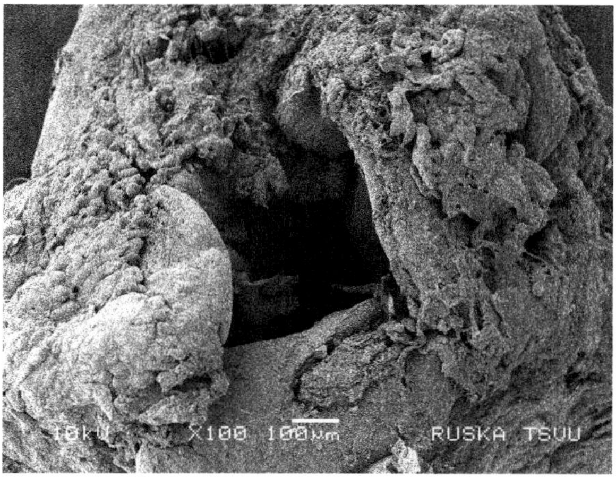

Fig. 4.3 Scanning electron microphotograph of the external surface of a punctum

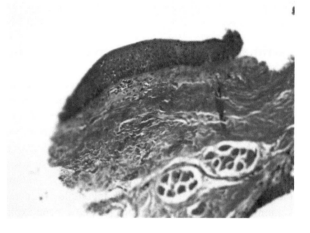

Fig. 4.4 Microphotograph showing pathological changes in punctal stenosis (Stain: Masson Trichrome, ×100)

muscle arrangement in the periphery of the canalicular walls and variably rugged external surfaces of the lacrimal system owing to crisscross arrangement of collagen bundles in lacrimal sac and nasolacrimal ducts (NLD) [7]. Presence of dense vascular plexus around lacrimal sac and NLD was noted similar to as shown by Paulsen et al. [8], which facilitates tear outflow via "wrung out" mechanism. No valvular areas were seen in NLD. Reasonably well discernable thickened junctional areas between inner-punctal surface–vertical canaliculus and lacrimal sac–NLD were noted, leading to a speculation about their possible functional roles. The exact role of these areas needs to be studied further, which might help further with etiopathogenesis of NLD obstructions (NLDO).

Etiopathogenesis of Punctal Stenosis

Punctal stenosis is one of the commonly encountered etiologies of epiphora, but its exact pathogenic mechanism is elusive as of now. A step toward unraveling its etiopathogenesis was attempted where immuno-phenotyping and electron microscopy of puncta was performed (Fig. 4.4) [9]. Infiltration of CD45+ and CD3+ T

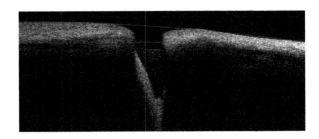

Fig. 4.5 Ocular coherence tomography image depicting the punctum and the vertical canaliculus

lymphocytes, focal B cell and plasma cell immunoreactivity along with numerous fibroblasts were the significant findings. Electron microscopy showed blunting of epithelial microvilli, abundant fibroblasts, disorderly arranged collagen bundles and mononuclear infiltration in the vicinity of fibroblasts or in between collagen bundles. The presence of specific T lymphocytes in the vicinity of fibroblasts had led to speculation about the possible role of immune cells rather than fibroblasts in triggering the events leading to punctal stenosis.

Lacrimal System Ocular Coherence Tomography

Proximal lacrimal system imaging using Fourier-domain optical coherence tomography (OCT) questioned the long-standing belief that the length of vertical canaliculus is 2 mm long. Maximal visualized depth of vertical canaliculus across published literature on OCT was 1400 μm with an average of 890 μm (Fig. 4.5) [10]. Imaging with spectralis using EDI technology has been found to be of prognostic value in punctal disorders like punctal stenosis, thereby helping in better preoperative counseling [11]. In addition, OCT features of numerous disorders of the proximal lacrimal system like incomplete punctal canalization [12], punctal keratin cyst [13], and canaliculops [14] have been explored recently.

Mitomycin C

Mitomycin C (MMC) has been used extensively in dacryocystorhinostomy (DCR) surgery; however, the appropriate concentrations and duration have not been standardized. A concentration of 0.2 mg/mL for 3 min was noted to inhibit the proliferation of human nasal mucosal fibroblasts without inducing apoptosis [15] and also correlated with in vitro collagen contractility and wound simulation [16] and hence was considered as an appropriate dose and duration in dacryocystorhinostomy surgeries (Fig. 4.6) [15]. Clinically, wound healing in the postoperative ostium is mediated by several cell types and occurs over a period of 6–8 weeks. Maintenance dose of MMC during healing period can be attained with injectable rather than topical application of MMC. Hence a newer technique of using Circumostial MMC injection in DCR at defined time-points have been proposed, which resulted in anatomical success of 89% in revision DCR (93% after one repeat surgery) and 97% in combined primary DCR and complex cases [17]. These

Fig. 4.6 Effect of mitomycin C (MMC) on fibroblast. The image shows the Phalloidin-DAPI merge image of cellular proliferation arrest with the use of MMC

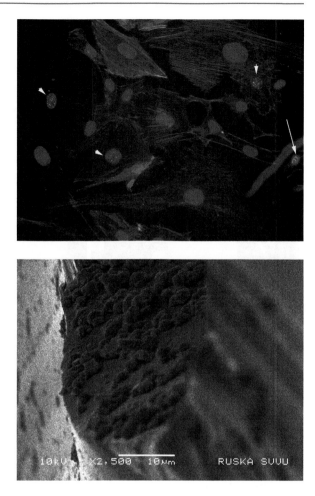

Fig. 4.7 Scanning electron microscopic image of a surface of lacrimal stent showing biofilms

effects were maintained in long-term assessments as well [18]. Transmission electron microscopic studies later confirmed the beneficial effects of both topical and COS MMC on the nasal mucosal healing, hence having implications in healing following dacryocystorhinostomy [19].

Lacrimal Stents

The great debate for and against stent usage in DCR surgeries is still unsettled. However, many surgeons agree upon selective intubation for canalicular stenosis, revision DCR, prolong surgeries, poor flaps and post-acute dacryocystitis. Bio-films have recently been studied on the external and luminal surfaces of extubated stents (Fig. 4.7) [20–23]. Biofilms were noted to be significant beyond 4 weeks of intubation. This combined with the data on postoperative ostium healing [24] suggests that stents, when used in lacrimal surgeries, should ideally not be kept beyond 4 weeks. In addition, extensive deposits and thick mixed biofilms constituted by fungal

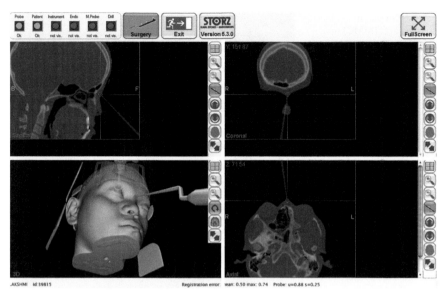

Fig. 4.8 Intraoperative image of an infrared navigation guidance

filaments and bacteria were found within the lumen and this led to a speculation about the possible benefits with the use of non-luminal stents.

Image Guided Lacrimal Surgeries

Complex SALDOs with distorted facial anatomy pose a difficult surgical challenge. Stereotactic navigation facilitates safe and precise dacryolocalization in such cases (Fig. 4.8) [25]. Imaging data is acquired preoperatively in the form of 3D CT/MRI and built into the navigation system, which then can be used for radio-anatomic correlation during surgery. Successful outcomes have been demonstrated in all complex cases in one of the series using Stealth navigation system [26, 27]. Newer introductions like telescopes enabled navigation, use of continuously variable viewing telescopes (Endochameleon) have transformed the endoscopic lacrimal surgeries [27, 28].

I-131 and NLDO

The reported frequency of NLDO ranges from 3.4% to 11% following iodine therapy [29]. Radio-uptake studies showed a significant intranasal localization of I-131 in patients receiving dose more than 150 millicurie (mCi) [30]. This could possibly reflect the underlying etiology for bilateral acquired NLDO observed in these cases. Screening of all patients (pre- and post-I-131 therapy), specifically those who receive a dose of more than 150 mCi should be performed. A screening protocol is now in place for patients receiving I-131 along with their risk stratification and clinical assessments [29].

Lacrimal Piezosurgery

The advent of ultrasonic bone emulsification in neurosurgery helped multiple subspecialties to explore this option. Ultrasonic endoscopic DCR has been explored as an alternative modality of managing NLD obstructions [31]. It was found to be safe and effective in both adult and pediatric populations and surgical outcomes were comparable to that of regular powered endoscopic DCRs [32]. In addition, it was also found that the time taken for superior osteotomy with the help of piezo techniques is not significantly different from that of mechanical drills [33]. There is also evidence to suggest that this may be a better modality to use for training in endoscopic DCR as compared to mechanical drills in view of its safety even in the hands of beginners.

Three-Dimensional (3D) Endoscopic Lacrimal Surgeries

The recent development of a 3D enabled 4 mm rigid telescope for nasal surgeries has the potential to revolutionize the way we perform endoscopic lacrimal surgeries (Fig. 4.9). Operating lacrimal surgeries like probing and DCR in 3D planes was found to enhance depth perception, dexterity, and precision compared with the routine 2D intraoperative views [34]. The surgical observers noted enhanced anatomical and surgical understandings in 3D compared with the 2D views [34]. Further detailed comparisons would help formulate guidelines for the routine use of 3D endoscopy in lacrimal surgeries.

Quality of Life in Lacrimal Disorders

There is an increasing shift from surgeon-reported outcomes to patient-reported outcomes in lacrimal disorders and quality of life (QOL) assessment is an essential outcome measure. Numerous QOL questionnaires like the Holmes, Glasgow benefit inventory, NLDO-symptom score (NLDO-SS), and lacrimal symptom scores (Lac-Q) are available. The use of Lac-Q is simple and reliable and has specific components addressing the lacrimal symptoms and social symptoms in brief [35]. The usefulness of Lac-Q has been studied in assessing the outcomes of powered endoscopic DCR and monoka stent dilatation for punctal stenosis which appears as a promising tool [36].

Fig. 4.9 The 3D-ORL Tipcam system for 3D nasal endoscopy

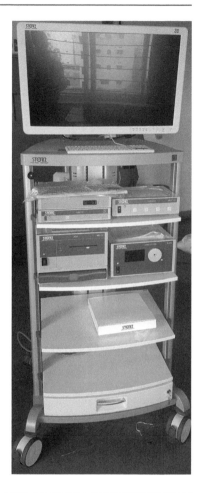

References

1. DeLancey JO. Current status of the subspecialty of female pelvic medicine and reconstructive surgery. Am J Obstet Gynecol. 2010;202:658.e1–4.
2. Vohra S, Surette S, Mittra D, et al. Pediatric integrative medicine: pediatrics' newest subspecialty? BMC Pediatr. 2012;12:123.
3. Shields JA, Shields CL. The development of ocular oncology. Watching a dream come true. Asia Pac J Ophthalmol (Phila). 2017;6:107–8.
4. Ali MJ. Principles and practice of lacrimal surgery. 2nd ed. New Delhi: Springer; 2017.
5. Ali MJ. Atlas of lacrimal drainage disorders. 1st ed. New Delhi: Springer; 2017.
6. Ali MJ, Schicht M, Paulsen F. Qualitative hormonal profiling of the lacrimal drainage system: potential insights into the etiopathogenesis of primary acquired nasolacrimal duct obstruction. Ophthal Plast Reconstr Surg. 2017;33(5):381–8. (Epub).
7. Ali MJ, Baig F, Lakshman M, Naik MN. Scanning electron microscopic features of the external and internal surfaces of normal adult lacrimal drainage system. Ophthal Plast Reconstr Surg. 2015;31:414–7.
8. Paulsen FP, Thale AB, Hallmann UJ, et al. The cavernous body of the human efferent tear ducts: function in tear outflow mechanism. Invest Ophthalmol Vis Sci. 2000;41:965–70.

 9. Ali MJ, Mishra DK, Baig F, Lakshman M, Naik MN. Punctal stenosis: histopathology, immunology, and electron microscopic features—a step toward unraveling the mysterious etiopathogenesis. Ophthal Plast Reconstr Surg. 2015;31:98–102.
10. Kamal S, Ali MJ, Ali MH, Naik MN. Fourier domain optical coherence tomography with 3D and en face imaging of the punctum and vertical canaliculus: a step towards establishing a normative database. Ophthal Plast Reconstr Surg. 2016;32:170–3.
11. Timlin HM, Keane PA, Rose GE, Ezra DG. Characterizing the occluded lacrimal punctum using anterior segment optical coherence tomography. Ophthal Plast Reconstr Surg. 2018;34(1):26–30. (Epub).
12. Singh S, Ali MJ, Naik MN. Familial incomplete punctal canalization: clinical and Fourier domain ocular coherence tomography features. Ophthal Plast Reconstr Surg. 2017;33:e66–9.
13. Kamal S, Ali MJ, Naik MN. Punctal keratinizing cyst: report in a pediatric patient with Fourier domain ocular coherence tomography features. Ophthal Plast Reconstr Surg. 2015;31:161–3.
14. Singh S, Ali MJ, Peguda H, et al. Imaging the caniculops with ultrasound biomicroscopy and anterior segment ocular coherence tomography. Ophthal Plast Reconstr Surg. 2017;33(6):e143–4. (Epub).
15. Ali MJ, Mariappan I, Maddileti S, et al. Mitomycin C in dacryocystorhinostomy: the search for the right concentration and duration—a fundamental study on human nasal mucosa fibroblasts. Ophthal Plast Reconstr Surg. 2013;29:469–74.
16. Kumar V, Ali MJ, Ramachandran C. Effect of mitomycin-C on contraction and migration of human nasal mucosal fibroblasts: implications in dacryocystorhinostomy. Br J Ophthalmol. 2015;99:1295–300.
17. Kamal S, Ali MJ, Naik MN. Circumostial injection of mitomycin C (COS-MMC) in external and endoscopic dacryocystorhinostomy: efficacy, safety profile, and outcomes. Ophthal Plast Reconstr Surg. 2014;30:187–90.
18. Singh M, Ali MJ, Naik MN. Long-term outcomes of circumostial injection of mitomycin C (COS-MMC) in dacryocystorhinostomy. Ophthal Plast Reconstr Surg. 2015;31:423–4.
19. Ali MJ, Baig F, Lakshman M, et al. Electron microscopic features of nasal mucosa treated with topical and circumostial injection of Mitomycin C: implications in dacryocystorhinostomy. Ophthal Plast Reconstr Surg. 2015;31:103–7.
20. Murphy J, Ali MJ, Psaltis AJ. Biofilm quantification on nasolacrimal silastic stents after dacryocystorhinostomy. Ophthal Plast Reconstr Surg. 2015;31:396–400.
21. Ali MJ, Baig F, Lakshman M, et al. Biofilms and physical deposits on nasolacrimal silastic stents following dacryocystorhinostomy: is there a difference between ocular and nasal segments? Ophthal Plast Reconstr Surg. 2015;31:452–5.
22. Ali MJ, Baig F, Lakshman M, et al. Scanning electron microscopic features of nasolacrimal silastic stents retained for prolong durations following dacryocystorhinostomy. Ophthal Plast Reconstr Surg. 2016;32:20–3.
23. Ali MJ, Baig F, Naik MN. Electron microscopic features of intraluminal portion of nasolacrimal silastic stents following dacryocystorhinostomy: is there a need for stents without a lumen? Ophthal Plast Reconstr Surg. 2016;32:252–6.
24. Ali MJ, Psaltis AJ, Ali MJ, et al. Endoscopic assessment of the dacryocystorhinostomy ostium after powered endoscopic surgery: behavior beyond 4 weeks. Clin Exp Ophthalmol. 2015;43:152–5.
25. Ali MJ, Naik MN. Image-guided dacryolocalization (IGDL) in traumatic secondary acquired lacrimal drainage obstructions (SALDO). Ophthal Plast Reconstr Surg. 2015;31:406–9.
26. Ali MJ, Singh S, Naik MN, Kaliki S, Dave TV. Interactive navigation-guided ophthalmic plastic surgery: the utility of 3D CT-DCG-guided dacryolocalization insecondary acquired lacrimal duct obstructions. Clin Ophthalmol. 2016;11:127–33.
27. Ali MJ, Singh S, Naik MN, Kaliki S, Dave TV. Interactive navigation-guidedophthalmic plastic surgery: navigation enabling of telescopes and their use inendoscopic lacrimal surgeries. Clin Ophthalmol. 2016;10:2319–24.
28. Ali MJ, Singh S, Naik MN. The usefulness of continuously variable view rigid endoscope in lacrimal surgeries: first intraoperative experience. Ophthal Plast Reconstr Surg. 2016;32:477–80.

29. Ali MJ. Iodine-131 therapy and nasolacrimal duct obstructions: what we know and what we need to know. Ophthal Plast Reconstr Surg. 2016;32:243–8.
30. Ali MJ, Vyakaranam AR, Rao JE, et al. Iodine-131 therapy and lacrimal drainage system toxicity: nasal localization studies using whole body nuclear scintigraphy and SPECT-CT. Ophthal Plast Reconstr Surg. 2017;33:13–6.
31. Ali MJ. Ultrasonic endoscopic dacryocystorhinostomy. In: Ali MJ, editor. Principles and practice of lacrimal surgery. New Delhi: Springer; 2015. p. 203–12.
32. Ali MJ, Singh M, Chisty N, et al. Endoscopic ultrasonic dacryocystorhinostomy: clinical profiles and outcomes. Eur Arch Otorhinolaryngol. 2016;273:1789–93.
33. Ali MJ, Ganguly A, Ali MJ, et al. Time taken for superior osteotomy in primary powered endoscopic dacryocystorhinostomy: is there a difference between an ultrasonic aspirator and a mechanical burr? Int Forum Allergy Rhinol. 2015;5:764–7.
34. Ali MJ, Naik MN. First intraoperative experience with three-dimensional (3D), high-definition nasal endoscopy for lacrimal surgeries. Eur Arch Otorhinolaryngol. 2017;274:2161–4.
35. Ali MJ. Quality of life in lacrimal disorders and patient satisfaction following management. In: Ali MJ, editor. Principles and practice of lacrimal surgery. New Delhi: Springer; 2015. p. 359–62.
36. Ali MJ, Iram S, Ali MH, et al. Assessing the outcomes of powered endoscopic DCR in adults using the lacrimal symptom (lac-Q) questionnaire. Ophthal Plast Reconstr Surg. 2017;33:65–8.

Advances in the Management of Orbital and Adnexal Trauma

5

Bipasha Mukherjee, Md Shahid Alam,
and Anantanarayanan Parameswaran

Introduction

Orbital fractures are common sequelae of cranio-maxillofacial trauma. The orbital bones can be fractured either in isolation or as a component of complex mid-facial or upper facial injury. Therefore, orbital fractures are classified depending upon the area involved [1, 2].

The orbit contains the globe and associated neurovascular complex that may get damaged in a traumatic event. Management of orbital and mid-facial fractures requires detailed ophthalmic evaluation, clinical examination of face and appropriate imaging [2].

High-resolution, three-dimensional (3D) formats and multi-planar, thin-cut (0.6 and 1 mm), computed tomography (CT) scans, augmented with 3D reconstruction, has revolutionized the preoperative evaluation of the surgical field (Fig. 5.1) [3].

B. Mukherjee (✉)
Orbit, Oculoplasty, Reconstructive and Aesthetic Services, Sankara Nethralaya,
Chennai, Tamil Nadu, India
e-mail: drbpm@snmail.org

M. S. Alam
Orbit, Oculoplasty, Reconstructive and Aesthetic Services, Sankara Nethralaya,
Kolkata, India

A. Parameswaran
Department of Oral and Maxillofacial Surgery, Meenakshiammal Dental College and
Hospital, Chennai, Tamil Nadu, India

© Springer Nature Singapore Pte Ltd. 2019
A. Gupta, P. Tahiliani (eds.), *Orbit and Oculoplastics*, Current Practices in
Ophthalmology, https://doi.org/10.1007/978-981-13-8538-4_5

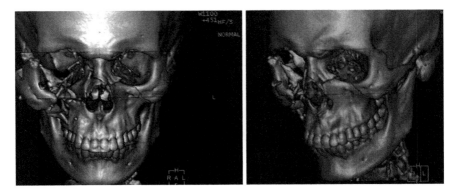

Fig. 5.1 Three-dimensional (3D) CT scan showing a displaced right ZMC fracture

Advances in Orbital Imaging

Reconstruction of the orbito-facial region is a challenge due to its complex anatomy, wide variety of available implants and associated cosmetic and psycho-social impact.

The principle goal of management of orbital trauma is different from the rest of the facial skeleton as more weightage is given to the restoration of intra-orbital volume than in restitution of the fractured fragments to their anatomical position. Integration of different technologies, such as preoperative computer-assisted planning for defining and simulating the desired outcome, intraoperative surgical navigation/CT scans, customized stereolithographic (STL) models have opened new avenues in the surgeons' armamentarium to tailor the reconstruction [4].

Stereolithography

The stereolithography (STL) was first used for planning a craniofacial surgery by Brix and Lambrecht in 1985 [4]. The data is recorded in a generic digital imaging and communications in medicine (DICOM) format and transferred to a Windows-based computer workstation with computer-assisted design (CAD) and computer-assisted manufacturing (CAM) software. The software converts the data for three-dimensional (3D) reconstruction in the axial, coronal, and sagittal views. 3D printer scan reads and analyzes the CT scan data and creates customized surgical models using a mirroring technique. Implants are then manufactured by subtractive manufacturing (machining a block of material) or by additive manufacturing (by adding material layer by layer and fusion of the layers).

Custom implants: Stereolithography models have proven beneficial in a wide range of surgical subspecialties. In cases of complex orbital trauma, STL offers

Fig. 5.2 Rapid prototype model of a patient, in which a model surgery has been performed and the ZMC has been optimally repositioned to facilitate pre-contouring of fixation implants

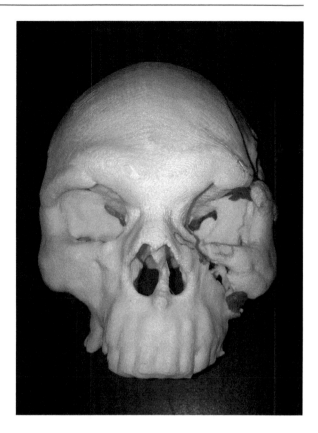

distinct advantages. Orbital implants were pre-formed based on the topographical analysis of the orbital cavity for the improvement of primary orbital reconstruction (Fig. 5.2) [5]. The concept is continuously evolving with advancements in the design, implant bio-materials and manufacturing processes [6]. These customized models can be sterilized and used in the operating room. Bending the plates on rapid prototyping models prior to the surgery reduces working time, thus preventing potential complications due to prolonged operative times. Further advancements in computer software and materials will lead to development of models of greater accuracy and lower cost, thus increasing their use in cases requiring complex post traumatic orbital reconstruction [7].

Virtual surgical planning: Preoperative computer-assisted virtual surgical planning (VSP) with virtual correction and construction of stereolithographic models have been used in conjunction with intraoperative navigation for precise reconstruction of the bony orbit. Such models may not be necessary for small orbital blowout fractures, but are promising for complex orbital trauma resulting in severe disruption or in secondary orbital reconstructions [8].

Intraoperative Navigation

Intraoperative navigation (ION) has its roots in neurosurgery and has been adapted from the standard usage of stereotaxy for neurosurgical procedures. The use of navigation assisted surgery in the head and neck region started in the late 1990s and gained much popularity in Europe in the early 2000s.

Key areas where ION may be indicated for orbital trauma (primary and secondary corrections) are:

1. Orbital floor reconstruction
2. Fractures of the zygomatico-maxillary complex (ZMC) and arch which are difficult to assess three dimensionally

Principles of Intraoperative Navigation

1. *Preoperative preparation*: the patient is prepared for ION with due considerations for the following:
   - CT scan or magnetic resonance imaging (MRI) which is taken according to the navigation protocol with no gantry shift
   - Preoperative planning of the surgical procedure
   - Determining the placement and position of the navigation sensor on the patient (typically a skull post; Fig. 5.3)
   - Completion of patient registration (Fig. 5.4) to calibrate the patient physically to the pre-loaded CT or MRI in the navigation console
2. *Planning for the surgical procedure:* This can be performed by two methods. The simpler method of mirroring (Fig. 5.5) can be performed if the correction required is unilateral. Here, the normal contralateral side is mirrored and fused with the deformed side which provides a template for the surgeon to compare and work intraoperatively. However, if the correction required is bilateral, the

Fig. 5.3 Fixing of navigation sensor on the patient's skull

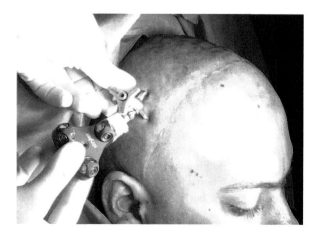

Fig. 5.4 Patient registration

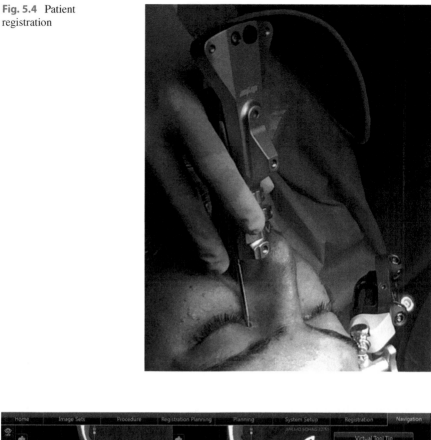

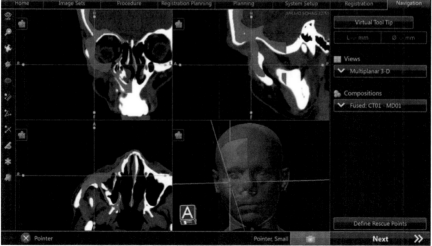

Fig. 5.5 Mirroring technique for virtual surgical planning

planning required is more demanding and it requires a segmentation and virtual surgery setup wherein the proposed correction is carried out virtually on a computer and the generated surgical plan is transferred into the navigation console in a recognizable digital format and fused with the patients current CT/MRI images.

3. *Patient registration*: The patient is physically registered and calibrated to the CT image by a face mask registration which is automatic or a manual registration where pre-determined points on the CT are calibrated by manual positioning of the navigation probe on the patient and registering them. Once the registration is completed, the position of the navigation probe on the patient is reflected as a virtual pointer on the pre-loaded patient images on the console thus displaying the virtual position for guidance.

Navigational surgery has improved the predictability of outcomes. Additionally, reconstruction abilities of the software can be used for virtual display of the patient's anatomy throughout the procedure, allowing stereotactic navigation. Computerized navigation consists of a virtual interface between the intraoperative positions of the surgical instruments with the reconstruction of patient anatomy, obtained by CT scans. In unilateral defects, navigation facilitates the procedure through mirroring techniques, and in bilateral defects, it imports virtual models from the standard CT datasets.

Intraoperatively, the navigation system controls the position of the implants or the mobilized bone and verifies the final location, thus reducing the element of human error. Intraoperative navigation enhances surgeons' ability to identify important anatomical landmarks to measure the extent of defect and to confirm the orientation of implants. It reduces the incidence of surgical complications due to improper orientation or position of plates and screws, and helps achieve a greater adherence to the preoperative plan [9].

These advances improve the efficiency, accuracy and safety of the surgical management of orbital trauma (Figs. 5.6 and 5.7).

Advances in Implant Materials and Designs Used in Orbital Trauma

An ideal implant for orbital fracture repair should be biocompatible, flexible, strong, preferably resorbable, and easily available at affordable price. An ideal implant remains elusive, and over the past 50 years, a number of substances have been tested to find the perfect material.

Traditionally, autologous bone grafts have been considered the gold standard for the repair of orbital floor fractures, owing to their inherent property of strength, vascularization and above all, their excellent biocompatibility [10]. Calvarial bone is considered to be the best option. Nevertheless, the drawbacks of autologous implants are considerable. The bone grafts are notoriously difficult to contour according to the defect, and excessive bending of graft beyond its natural capacity can break it. The resorption rates are unpredictable and may vary over a wide duration. Last but not the least is the donor site morbidity. The following table summarizes the available implants with their salient features:

Type	Material	Commercial name	Comment
Bioceramics	Hydroxyapatite (HA)		Expensive, fibrovascular growth
	Bioactive glass		Promotes osteogenesis along the implant
Metals	Titanium	MatrixORBITAL	Fibrosis, orbital soft tissue adherence
	Cobalt alloys	Vitallium	Rarely used, artifacts on CT making it difficult to image pathologies
Polymer	Polyethylene (PE)	Medpor	Commonly used, expensive
	Polytetraflouroethylene (PTFE)	Gore-Tex	
	Nylon	Suprafoil	
	Polylactic acid (PLA)	Biosorb	Bioabsorbable
	Polyglycolic acid (PGA)	LactoSorb	
	Polyetheretherketone (PEEK)		Custom implants; used in craniofacial defects
Composites	HA/PE	HAPEX	
	Titanium/PE	Medpor Titan	
	PLA and PGA, polydioxanone (PDO)		Ideal in pediatric population

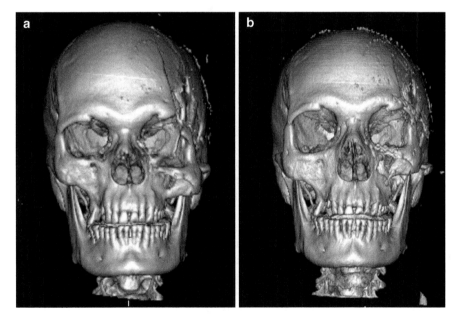

Fig. 5.6 CT scan showing left zygomatico-maxillary complex fracture with concomitant left cranial defect

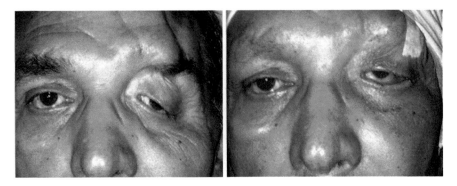

Fig. 5.7 Preoperative enophthalmos and inferior dystopia seen. Patient underwent reoconstruction of the left ZMC with pre-contoured implants with cranial defect closure by coronal, intra-oral vestibular and transconjunctival approach along with osteotomy along the supraorbital rim, zygomatic arch and infraorbital rim. The left zygomatico-maxillary complex (ZMC) was fractured and mobilized superiorly and medially and fixed with precontoured implants and screws. Postoperatively, residual enophthalmos of 2 mm seen with good correction

Based on the risks and benefits of the inherent properties of the implants, the best suited can be used.

Management of Traumatic Nasolacrimal Duct Obstruction

The incidence of traumatic nasolacrimal duct obstructions (TrNLDO) has increased in recent years due to increasing number of road traffic accidents. The nasolacrimal duct (NLD) lies in the lateral nasal wall and any trauma to the mid-face and resulting naso-orbital-ethmoid (NOE) fracture can cause TrNLDO.

The distorted anatomy secondary to the NOE fractures and pre-existing plates and screws from previous facio-maxillary interventions renders the management of this condition challenging. Management of traumatic NLDO has seen a few advances which can be elaborated as follows.

1. **Computerized dacryocystography (CT-DCG):** Dacryocystography is done in cases of TrNLDO to locate the site of obstruction and the actual location of lacrimal sac. Earlier, for DCG, a contrast medium was injected into the lacrimal system via syringe and the radiologist usually needed an ophthalmologist to carry out the procedure. The procedure has become much simpler with the advent of radio-opaque drops which are instilled in the conjunctival cul de sac and the whole lacrimal system can be imaged after few seconds [11, 12]. The drops are prepared by diluting the iohexol contrast agent with distilled water in a 1:1 dilution [12].Freitag et al. were first to describe CT-DCG in 2002 and the

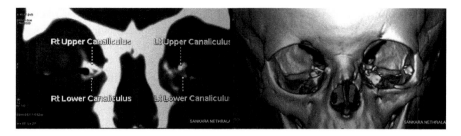

Fig. 5.8 CT-DCG

procedure has since gained popularity among surgeons managing lacrimal system trauma [13]. The cone beam CT used routinely by the oral surgeons offers added advantage of the imaging being done in the anatomic position with the patient being seated. CT-DCG demonstrates the lacrimal drainage system and its relationship with the surrounding bony structures (Fig. 5.8). The 3D reconstruction of CT-DCG can also be utilized for localization in navigation guided lacrimal surgery, especially in cases where routine bony landmarks are not available for guiding the surgery [14].The thin slice helical CT with 2D and 3D reconstructions offers excellent image resolution and preoperative planning. TrNLDO can be routinely managed by dacryocystorhinostomy (DCR) with excellent success. Mukherjee et al. reported 96% success rate in their series [15]. The preferred approach is external in such cases; however, endoscopic nasal route is also being increasingly utilized with good outcomes [15–17].

2. **Endoscopes:** Managing traumatic NLDO via endoscopic nasal route is still challenging because of the distorted anatomy and limited nasal space in many of these cases. Following modifications of the endoscopes have made this approach simpler and easier.

  (a) *Variable view rigid endoscope*: The current endoscopes have a fixed viewing angle (0°, 30°, 45°, 70° or 90°) and working distance. A continuous variable view camera tip can enable the view over a wide range of angles in one plane without the need to move the endoscope intraoperatively. The modification allows the entire extent of sac and surrounding structures to be visualized in much more detail without the need for changing telescopes every time and can be very helpful in cases of traumatic NLDO [18].

  (b) *Three-dimensional endoscope*: Current rigid endoscopes provide a two-dimensional view and hence lack depth perception. The 3D endoscope is a recently launched newer generation endoscope which can be very useful with enhanced stereopsis [19].

  (c) *Navigation enabled endoscope*: Routine navigation requires the navigation seeker to be placed at multiple anatomical points for multiple times. The problem can be circumvented if the tip of endoscope itself can be used as a navigation seeker. The navigation enabled endoscope provides this option and is a very useful addition to the navigation guided surgery in managing these complex cases [20].

3. **Image-guided dacryolocalization:** Image-guided surgery was first described by Horseley and Clarke [21]. Ali et al. coined the term "image guided dacryolocalization," in which they used the navigation system for managing a case of complex TrNLDO [22].

4. **Mitomycin C (MMC):** Scarring and cicatricial closure of the ostium are the most common causes for failure of external DCR. Postoperative inflammation and scarring can be far more extensive in patients of trauma resulting in failure of DCR. MMC has been advocated as an adjunct to DCR to prevent fibrosis, and thus, failure. It has been used in varying concentrations ranging from 0.05 to 0.5 mg/mL for durations ranging from 2 to 15 min. Ali et al. studied the effects of MMC on nasal mucosa fibroblasts and found that the minimum effective concentration was 0.2 mg/mL for 3 min [23]. In order to achieve higher drug concentration for prolonged duration, they also suggested circumostial injection of MMC 0.02% at four different sites [24].

5. **Intubation:** Intubation of the lacrimal system after a primary or revision DCR has been a popular adjunct to the surgery in the hope of preventing scarring along the path of the stent. DCR after TrNLDO is commonly supplemented with silicone intubation; however, the duration for which the stent should be retained has been debated. Previously, the stent used to be in place for as long as 12 weeks; however, recent studies suggest no added advantage beyond 4 weeks of duration [25]. Systematic review and meta-analysis on the effect of silicone intubation in cases of primary NLDO suggest no added advantage with similar success rates with or without stenting, the same, however, remains to be proven for TrNLDO [26, 27].

In conclusion, management of orbital trauma and complex nasolacrimal duct obstructions has advanced in leaps and bounds in recent years. Recent advancements in surgical as well as imaging techniques have considerably improved both the functional and esthetic outcomes of orbital reconstruction.

References

1. Kunz C, Audigé L, Cornelius C-P, Buitrago-Téllez C, Rudderman R, Prein J. The comprehensive AOCMF classification system: orbital fractures—level 3 tutorial. Craniomaxillofac Trauma Reconstr. 2014;7:S092–102.
2. Kashima T. Types and management of orbital fractures. In: Mukherjee B, Yuen H, editors. Emergencies of the orbit and adnexa. New Delhi: Springer; 2017. p. 95–9. http://link.springer.com/10.1007/978-81-322-1807-4_14.
3. Holck DE, Boyd EM, Ng J, Mauffray RO. Benefits of stereolithography in orbital reconstruction. Ophthalmology. 1999;106:1214–8.
4. Bell RB, Markiewicz MR. Computer-assisted planning, stereolithographic modeling, and intraoperative navigation for complex orbital reconstruction: a descriptive study in a preliminary cohort. J Oral Maxillofac Surg. 2009;67:2559–70.
5. Herford AS, Miller M, Lauritano F, Cervino G, Signorino F, Maiorana C. The use of virtual surgical planning and navigation in the treatment of orbital trauma. Chin J Traumatol. 2017;20:9–13.
6. Malyala SK, Kumar RY. A review on rapid prototyping technologies in biomedical applications. Int J Recent Sci Res. 2016;7:10783–9.

7. Sinn DP, Cillo JE, Miles BA. Stereolithography for craniofacial surgery. J Craniofac Surg. 2006;17:869–75.
8. Beigi B, McMullan TFW, Gupta D, Khandwala M. Stereolithographic models to guide orbital and oculoplastic surgery. Graefes Arch Clin Exp Ophthalmol. 2010;248:551–4.
9. Novelli G, Tonellini G, Mazzoleni F, Bozzetti A, Sozzi D. Virtual surgery simulation in orbital wall reconstruction: integration of surgical navigation and stereolithographic models. J Cranio-Maxillofac Surg. 2014;42:2025–34.
10. Schlickewei W, Schlickewei C. The use of bone substitutes in the treatment of bone defects—the clinical view and history. Macromol Symp. 2007;253:10–23. https://doi.org/10.1002/masy.200750702.
11. Manfrè L, de Maria M, Todaro E, Mangiameli A, Ponte F, Lagalla R. MR dacryocystography: comparison with dacryocystography and CT dacryocystography. AJNR Am J Neuroradiol. 2000;21:1145–50.
12. Udhay P, Noronha OV, Mohan RE. Helical computed tomographic dacryocystography and its role in the diagnosis and management of lacrimal drainage system blocks and medial canthal masses. Indian J Ophthalmol. 2008;56:31–7.
13. Freitag SK, Woog JJ, Kousoubris PD, Curtin HD. Helical computed tomographic dacryocystography with three-dimensional reconstruction: a new view of the lacrimal drainage system. Ophthal Plast Reconstr Surg. 2002;18:121–32.
14. Ali MJ, Singh S, Naik MN, Kaliki S, Dave TV. Interactive navigation-guided ophthalmic plastic surgery: the utility of 3D CT-DCG-guided dacryolocalization in secondary acquired lacrimal duct obstructions. Clin Ophthalmol. 2016;11:127–33.
15. Mukherjee B, Dhobekar M. Traumatic nasolacrimal duct obstruction: clinical profile, management, and outcome. Eur J Ophthalmol. 2013;23:615–22.
16. Ali MJ, Gupta H, Honavar SG, Naik MN. Acquired nasolacrimal duct obstructions secondary to naso-orbito-ethmoidal fractures: patterns and outcomes. Ophthal Plast Reconstr Surg. 2012;28(4):242–5.
17. Uzun F, Karaca EE, Konuk O. Surgical management of traumatic nasolacrimal duct obstruction. Eur J Ophthalmol. 2016;26(6):517–9.
18. Ali MJ, Singh S, Naik MN. The usefulness of continuously variable view rigid endoscope in lacrimal surgeries: first intraoperative experience. Ophthal Plast Reconstr Surg. 2016;32(6):477–80.
19. Ali MJ, Naik MN. First intraoperative experience with three-dimensional (3D) high-definition (HD) nasal endoscopy for lacrimal surgeries. Eur Arch Otorhinolaryngol. 2017;274(5):2161–4.
20. Ali MJ, Singh S, Naik MN, Kaliki S, Dave TV. Interactive navigation-guided ophthalmic plastic surgery: navigation enabling of telescopes and their use in endoscopic lacrimal surgeries. Clin Ophthalmol. 2016;10:2319–24.
21. Fodstad H, Hariz M, Ljunggren B. History of Clarke's stereotactic instrument. Stereotact Funct Neurosurg. 1991;57:130–40.
22. Ali MJ, Naik MN. Image-guided dacryolocalization (IGDL) in traumatic secondary acquired lacrimal drainage obstructions (SALDO). Ophthal Plast Reconstr Surg. 2015;31(5):406–9.
23. Ali MJ, Mariappan I, Maddileti S, et al. Mitomycin C in dacryocystorhinostomy: the search for the right concentration and duration—a fundamental study on human nasal mucosa fibroblasts. Ophthal Plast Reconstr Surg. 2013;29:469–74.
24. Kamal S, Ali MJ, Naik MN. Circumostial injection of mitomycin C (COS-MMC) in external and endoscopic dacryocystorhinostomy: efficacy, safety profile, and outcomes. Ophthal Plast Reconstr Surg. 2014;30(2):187–90.
25. Ali MJ, Psaltis AJ, Ali MH, Wormald PJ. Endoscopic assessment of the dacryocystorhinostomy ostium after powered endoscopic surgery: behaviour beyond 4 weeks. Clin Exp Ophthalmol. 2015;43(2):152–5.
26. Sarode D, Bari DA, Cain AC. The benefit of silicone stents in primary endoscopic dacryocystorhinostomy: a systematic review and meta-analysis. Clin Otolaryngol. 2007;42:307–14.
27. Feng YF, Cai JQ, Zhang JY, Han XH. A meta-analysis of primary dacryocystorhinostomy with and without silicone intubation. Can J Ophthalmol. 2011;46:521–7.

Periocular Rejuvenation: A Brief Overview

6

Prerana Tahiliani and Adit Gupta

Introduction

Periocular rejuvenation essentially consists of non-invasive rejuvenation and surgical rejuvenation. It may be indicated for the purpose of solely enhancing cosmesis or to rectify a complication of a prior cosmetic correction. Recent advances focus on minimally invasive scarless techniques in achieving this goal. Additionally, the use of dermal fillers has changed the way esthetic surgery is practiced.

Traditional rejuvenation involved more of surgery with removal of skin, muscle and fat from the eyelid tissues to achieve a lift or reduce laxity. Over a period of time, the concept of aging has changed with deflation being considered as a major factor in redundancy of tissues [1]. Excessive removal of skin and soft tissue often leads to hollow and unnatural looking eyelids [2]. Sometimes it can lead to inadequate closure of the eyelids leading to ocular surface complications.

Evaluation of the Cosmetic Patient

In esthetic practice, evaluation and counseling are more important than the procedure itself. There are certain points which need to be taken into account while dealing with a patient demanding a cosmetic procedure.

- Evaluation of the skin color, quality, and texture.
- The eyelid-eyebrow complex as a whole.

P. Tahiliani (✉)
Mumbai Eye Plastic Surgery, Mumbai, Maharashtra, India

A. Gupta
Mumbai Eye Plastic Surgery, Mumbai, Maharashtra, India

Department of Ophthalmology, Deenanath Mangeshkar Hospital, Pune, Maharashtra, India

© Springer Nature Singapore Pte Ltd. 2019
A. Gupta, P. Tahiliani (eds.), *Orbit and Oculoplastics*, Current Practices in Ophthalmology, https://doi.org/10.1007/978-981-13-8538-4_6

61

- The differentiation of fat pocket from a fluid pocket. This can be achieved by asking the patient to look up and down. Fat pocket typically increases on upgaze and decreases on downgaze, while fluid pocket remains constant.
- Eyelid position, tone, and symmetry which include the presence of a lax eyelid.
- Ruling out borderline cases of body dysmorphic disorder.

After the initial consult, it is important to decide between surgical versus nonsurgical treatment options.

Noninvasive periocular rejuvenation includes:

1. Dermal filler injections
2. Botulinum toxin injections
3. Skin care regimen

Surgical periocular rejuvenation encompasses:

1. Upper eyelid blepharoplasty
2. Lower eyelid blepharoplasty
3. Correction of proptosis
4. Ptosis correction

Dermal Fillers for Periocular Hollowing

Periocular hollows develop along the ligamentous attachments between skin and bone and skin and muscle due to constant eyelid movement. For cases of under eye hollows and mild to moderate fat prolapse, an acceptable esthetic improvement can be achieved by using dermal fillers [3, 4]. This technique needs sound knowledge of eyelid and orbital anatomy to avoid complications and have minimal downtime (Figs. 6.1 and 6.2).

In this technique, a hyaluronic acid gel (HAG) filler is injected in a suitable amount based on the patient's facial profile. Appropriate patient selection and counseling is paramount and more determining than correct technique of injection.

Technique of Dermal Filler Injection

Injections are carried out under topical anesthesia (Lidocaine + Prilocaine) applied 30–60 min before the procedure. The injection site is cleaned and sterilized with alcohol immediately before the injection. Using a 30-gauge needle, the HAG is injected in the pre-periosteal plane deep to the orbicularis oculi muscle, using a feathering technique where layered distribution of the product is achieved. To minimize bruising, the needle is withdrawn all the way out through the skin only when needed to reposition for another series of passages. Quick, gentle, continuous pressure is applied as soon as the needle is withdrawn to avoid bruising. It is important to

Fig. 6.1 Pre and post 1 cc dermal filler for tear trough hollows. Note the improvement in the bony rim represented in the image as depicted by the arrow

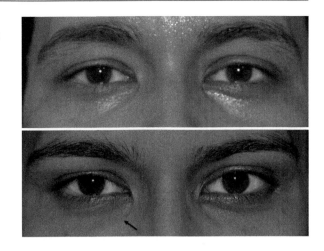

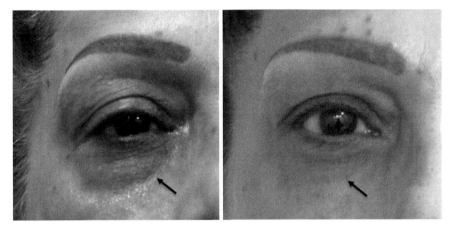

Fig. 6.2 Treatment of lower eyelid fat prolapse with dermal filler. Note the improvement of the contour of the lower eyelid–midface junction post procedure

avoid depositing large volumes of the filler in one location to prevent lumps and bumps. Superficial injection of the filler may cause visible bluish discoloration which may have to be dissolved at a later date.

Dermal fillers also have been used to volumize the eyebrows and give a three dimensional projection to the aging eyebrow fat pads [5].

Apart from purely cosmetic indications, dermal filler injections have also been used to correct eyelid malposition including entropion, epiblepharon, and eyelid retraction [6]. Asymmetric upper eyelid retraction in cases of thyroid eye disease can be corrected nonsurgically using HAG injections (Fig. 6.3). The placement of the gel in the levator plane is of utmost importance in these cases. We believe that there is a mechanical stretching of the levator muscle causing change in eyelid position.

Fig. 6.3 Correction of eyelid malposition with dermal fillers. This lady with inactive thyroid eyelid retraction received 1 cc hyaluronic acid gel filler injection in the left eyelid with immediate improvement as noted in the image

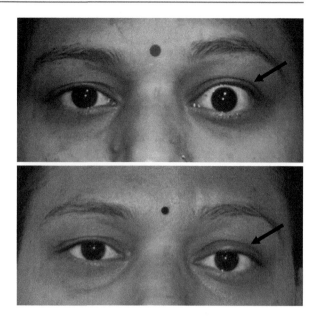

The longevity of dermal filler injections varies from 6 to 12 months depending on the product and the area injected [3]. There are some studies which mention the fillers lasting for more than 12 months in the periocular region.

Advantages of Dermal Fillers
1. Minimally invasive
2. Can be performed in the clinic
3. Can be reversed with hyaluronidase injections

Disadvantages
1. Expensive
2. Can cause fluid retention in some cases
3. Bluish discoloration if injected superficial—Tyndall phenomenon
4. Very rarely can cause vascular complications if injected within a vessel

Botulinum Toxin

Botulinum toxin has often been used by ophthalmologists for the treatment of blepharospasm and hemifacial spasm. Recently, it has gained importance for cosmetic treatments as well. For periocular rejuvenation, botulinum toxin injections can be used to treat dynamic rhytids arising from the repetitive contractions of the periocular muscles [7–9].

The most common cosmetic indications of botulinum toxin around the eyes are summarized in Table 6.1.

Table 6.1   Summarizes use of botulinum toxin in the periocular region

Indication	Target muscle	Dosage (units)	Remarks
Crow's feet (Fig. 6.4)	Lateral orbicularis	12–30 U varies according to muscle mass	Avoid injecting within the orbital rim Check for eyelid laxity prior to injection
Forehead lines	Frontalis	Women: 10–15 U Men: 20–25 U	Injection point should be at least 1–2 cm above the orbital rim to avoid eyebrow droop
Glabellar lines	Procerus, corrugator supercilii	Women: 20–25 U Men: 30–35 U	Consider interaction with frontalis muscle to avoid exaggerated peak of the lateral eyebrow
Bunny lines (Fig. 6.4)	Nasalis	2–4 U	This muscle needs minimal dosage

Fig. 6.4 Injection points for botulinum toxin in the crow's feet region (marked with black dots), bunny lines (marked with blue asterisk), and lower orbicularis roll (marked with red square)

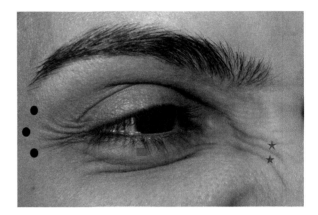

Lower Blepharoplasty

The lower eyelid comprises of three fat pads, the medial and the central separated by the inferior oblique muscle and the central and the lateral separated by the arcuate ligament. Knowing the anatomy of these fat pads is important before planning a blepharoplasty. Also, the distinction of fat from fluid is very important before performing any lower eyelid procedure. A simple test for this is to ask the patient look up and down while noticing the change in the lower eyelid. Fat usually becomes more prominent in upgaze and decreases in downgaze.

Lower eyelid blepharoplasty is one of the most commonly performed procedures by an oculoplastic surgeon. It has transitioned over time from anterior transcutaneous approach to the hidden transconjunctival approach via the fornix of the eyelid (Fig. 6.5). Nowadays, repositioning of the orbital fat pedicles onto the cheek is a favored procedure to augment the volume, avoid under eye hollowing, and achieve a smoother contour. The repositioning is done in the preperiosteal/subperiosteal plane, and all of this can be achieved via a hidden trans-conjunctival approach [10].

Fig. 6.5 Lower eyelid transconjunctival blepharoplasty (Image Courtesy: Dr. Robert Goldberg, UCLA). Pre- and postoperative images showing the improvement in the lower eyelid fat prolapse after a transconjunctival lower eyelid blepharoplasty

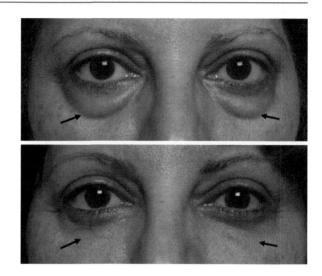

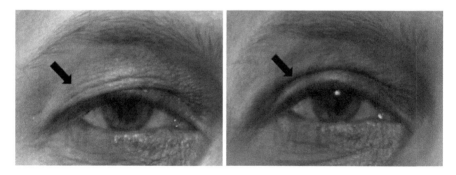

Fig. 6.6 Upper eyelid blepharoplasty. Pre- and post-surgery images of a patient with dermatochalasis who underwent upper eyelid blepharoplasty. Note the change in the appearance of the eyelid fold and the tarsal platform

Upper Blepharoplasty

Upper eyelid blepharoplasty is performed in patients with dermatochalasis who have a loose and hanging eyelid fold (Fig. 6.6). This procedure may be medically necessary in extreme cases where the eyelid fold obscures the visual axis.

The procedure can be performed as a day care surgery under local anesthesia. Depending on the severity, only skin or skin–muscle–fat excision is performed. The extent of excision depends on preoperative measurements. As a rule, approximately 20 mm height of eyelid skin has to be left after excision for adequate closure of the eyelid.

Upper eyelid blepharoplasty can be combined with adjunctive surgical procedures like lateral canthoplasty to tighten the lower eyelid, brassiere suture to enhance the eyebrow fat pad, medial fat pad removal to reduce the puffiness and lacrimal gland repositioning for prolapsed lacrimal gland [10]. All these procedures can be performed via the same incision and so are best done at the time of the initial surgery.

Correction of Proptosis

Thyroid eye disease (TED) is one of the most common causes of disfiguring proptosis leading to functional as well as cosmetic abnormalities. The disease follows the Rundle's curve consisting of an active inflammatory phase and a passive phase of subsiding inflammation. After the active phase of TED subsides, chronic sequelae remains which can be cosmetically disfiguring. There are various surgical options for the treatment of these sequelae which include orbital decompression for bulging eyes, levator recession surgery for retracted eyelids, and eyelid contouring eventually for cosmetic enhancement [11].

Thyroid decompression surgery can be performed via a keyhole approach using minimal incisions. A combination of external approach (incision through the eyelid/caruncle) and endonasal endoscopic approach for a better suited outcome has been made possible due to better understanding of the anatomy. We have shifted our focus to lateral wall and fat decompression as the preferred initial approaches to decompression surgery.

Eyelid retraction surgery in the form of levator recession and lower eyelid retractor recession can now be performed via the posterior approach avoiding an eyelid scar.

Ptosis Surgery

Droopy eyelid is a common cause of concern as it may impart a tired look. As we age, the eyelid tissues become lax and lead to dehiscence of the levator muscle aponeurosis which causes a droop of the upper lid. Traditionally, ptosis surgery was approached via the eyelid crease skin, but nowadays, posterior approach ptosis surgery can be offered avoiding an external scar [12] (Fig. 6.7). Mullerectomy surgery involves resecting a particular length of the conjunctiva and Muller's muscle complex which causes a shortening in the posterior lamella in turn lifting the eyelid [13]. There are various nomograms followed all over the world to determine the amount of resection needed. We follow a simple rule: for every 4 mm of conjunctiva resected, approximately 1 mm of eyelid lift is achieved.

When a ptosis surgery has to be combined with an upper eyelid blepharoplasty, the anterior eyelid crease approach is preferable as both the surgeries can be performed via the same incision.

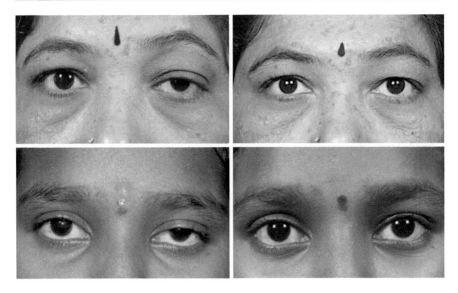

Fig. 6.7 Correction of ptosis. Upper image shows the correction of acquired aponeurotic ptosis with Mullers muscle conjunctival resection. Lower image shows congenital ptosis correction via an external levator resection approach

Conclusion

Ophthalmic plastic surgery for the periocular area needs a balance of skillful application of anatomical knowledge and the art of cosmesis. Often, these procedures can be combined with skin enhancing procedures, such as chemical peels and lasers to augment the esthetic outcome. Studying the details of each case profile and customizing the management is the key to a happy patient. We certainly do not have all the answers, which makes the field exciting for all the doctors practicing this subject to develop better techniques in the years to come.

References

1. Zimbler MS, Kokoska MS, Thomas JR. Anatomy and pathophysiology of facial aging. Facial Plast Surg Clin North Am. 2001;9:179–87.
2. Goldberg RA. Future of cosmetic surgery. Facial Plast Surg. 2014;30:101–2.
3. Goldberg RA, Fiaschetti D. Filling the periorbital hollows with hyaluronic acid gel: initial experience with 244 injections. Ophthalmic Plast Reconstr Surg. 2006;22:335–41.
4. Lambros VS. Hyaluronic acid injections for correction of the tear trough deformity. Plast Reconstr Surg. 2007;120:74–80.
5. Mustak H, Fiaschetti D, Gupta A, Goldberg R. Eyebrow contouring with hyaluronic acid gel filler injections. J Clin Aesthet Dermatol. 2018;11:38–40.
6. Taban M, Mancini R, Nakra T, Veez FG, Ela-Delman N, Tsirbas A, Douglas RS, Goldberg RA. Nonsurgical management of eyelid malposition using hyaluronic acid gel. Ophthalmic Plast Reconstr Surg. 2009;25(4):259–63.

7. Carruthers A, Carruthers J. Botulinum toxin type a for the treatment of glabellar rhytids. Dermatol Clin. 2004;22:137–44.
8. Carruthers J, Fagien S, Matarasso SL. Consensus recommendations on the use of botulinum toxin type a in facial aesthetics. Plast Reconstr Surg. 2004;114(6 suppl):1S–22S.
9. Olsen J. Balanced botox chemodenervation of the upper face: symmetry in motion. Semin Plast Surg. 2007;21(1):47–53.
10. Naik MN, Honavar SG, Dhepe N. Blepharoplasty: an overview. J Cutan Aesthet Surg. 2009;2(1):6–11.
11. Naik MN, Nair AG, Gupta A, Kamal S. Minimally invasive surgery for thyroid eye disease. Indian J Ophthalmol. 2015;63:847–53.
12. Allen RC, Saylor MA, Nerad JA. The current state of ptosis repair: a comparison of internal and external approaches. Curr Opin Ophthalmol. 2011;22:394–9.
13. Sajja K, Putterman AM. Mullers muscle conjunctival resection ptosis repair in the aesthetic patient. Saudi J Ophthalmol. 2011;25:51–60.

Emerging Trends in Socket Reconstruction

7

Kasturi Bhattacharjee and Andrea Tongbram

Introduction

An anophthalmic socket poses a challenge for the ophthalmologist and the ocularist, and causes significant psychological morbidity to the patient due to cosmetic aberrations and profound functional disturbances from the loss of an eye [1]. The reconstruction of anophthalmic socket requires meticulous surgical techniques to enable fitting of a cosmetically acceptable prosthetic eye along with adequate eyelid function.

An ideal anophthalmic socket should have the following characteristics [2]:

1. An orbital implant of adequate size which is central and well covered
2. Healthy conjunctival lining with well-formed and deep fornices
3. Normal tone and position of the eyelids including that of the eyelid margin
4. Satisfactory movement of overlying prosthesis over the implant

Contracted Socket

A contracted socket results from inadequate orbital volume or surface area of the conjunctiva or both.

Formation of a contracted socket may be attributed to failure of correction of congenital anophthalmos, microphthalmos and cystic ocular remnants. Among the acquired causes, inadequate sized orbital implant and conjunctival scarring due to

K. Bhattacharjee (✉)
Department of Ophthalmic Plastic Surgery, Sri Sankaradeva Nethralaya,
Guwahati, Assam, India

A. Tongbram
Department of Orbit, Oculoplasty and Reconstructive Services, Sankara Nethralaya,
Chennai, Tamil Nadu, India

© Springer Nature Singapore Pte Ltd. 2019
A. Gupta, P. Tahiliani (eds.), *Orbit and Oculoplastics*, Current Practices in
Ophthalmology, https://doi.org/10.1007/978-981-13-8538-4_7

trauma, excessive tissue handling and cauterization during surgery, chronic inflammation, infection, radiation and prior socket surgeries are the common causes.

Classification of Contracted Socket

Of the many classification systems proposed for contracted socket, the grading described by Krishna [3] is widely used.

Krishna classified contracted sockets into the following five grades:

- **Grade I**—shortening of the inferior fornix (Fig. 7.1)
- **Grade II**—shortening of both superior and inferior fornices (Fig. 7.2)
- **Grade III**—shortening of all four fornices (Fig. 7.3)
- **Grade IV**—Grade III + reduced vertical and horizontal palpebral aperture dimensions (Fig. 7.4)
- **Grade V**—recurrence of contracture after repeated trial of reconstruction

Examination of the Socket

Clinical evaluation of a socket entails assessment of the following features:

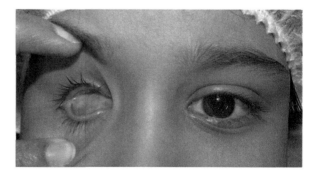

Fig. 7.1 Contracted socket right eye showing shortening of inferior fornix only (Grade I)

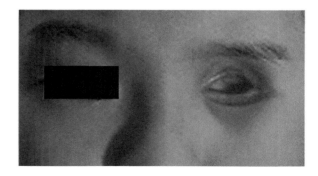

Fig. 7.2 Contracted socket left eye showing shortening of superior and inferior fornices (Grade II)

Fig. 7.3 Contracted
socket right eye showing
shortening of all four
fornices (Grade III)

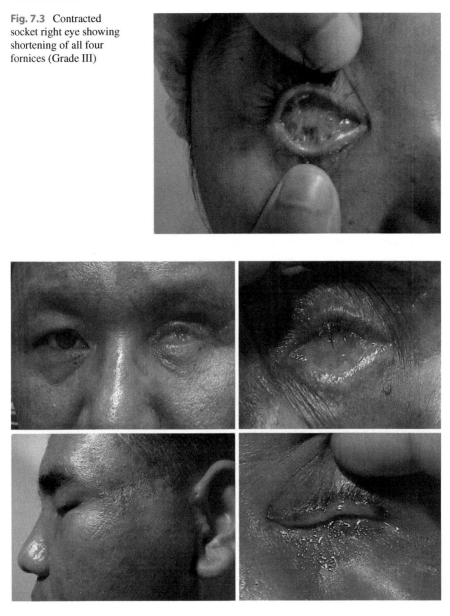

Fig. 7.4 Contracted socket left eye showing shortening of all four fornices + decrease in vertical
and horizontal palpebral aperture dimensions (Grade IV)

1. Surface area of the socket: Adequacy or inadequacy of the conjunctival surface
   and the depth of fornices are assessed.
2. Volume: A socket without an orbital implant or with a smaller sized implant has
   low orbital volume. This is sometimes compensated by a larger volume of

custom ocular prosthesis causing eyelid deformities. Superior sulcus deformity, entropion and ptosis are surrogates for reduced orbital volume.

3. Dry/wet socket: It is important to assess the health of the conjunctival epithelium and rule out granulomas and discharging sinuses.
4. Eyelid abnormalities like entropion, superior sulcus deformity and ptosis may be secondary to an inadequate implant volume or ill fitted prosthesis. Eyelid laxity, eyelid notches and lagophthalmos are also noted.
5. Associated bony deformities and contracture should be assessed particularly post radiotherapy.

Reconstruction of an Anophthalmic Socket

- Meticulous dissection during the primary surgery (evisceration/enucleation).
- Excessive conjunctival sacrifice or use of cautery should be avoided.
- Implant of adequate size and volume should be placed during the primary procedure as far as feasible.
- A conformer should always be placed at the end of the procedure till the placement of prosthesis. This keeps the conjunctival surface stretched and maintains the depth of the fornices.
- Custom ocular prosthesis of optimal size and contour and free of any irregularities on its surface should be placed after wound healing.

Management of Socket Contracture

Congenital Socket Contracture

This is seen in cases of congenital anophthalmos and microphthalmos. These patients have both soft tissue as well as bony contracture. The palpebral fissure is narrow both horizontally as well as vertically and there is deficiency of the palpebral and bulbar conjunctiva. The presence of normal sized globe is a prerequisite not only for the growth of the orbit and the lids but also for surrounding facial skeleton and the sinuses. The eye grows fastest in the first year of life with 70% of its adult size attained by 4 years, 90% by 7 years and completed by 14 years of age [4–6]. Management of these patients should include a stepwise approach involving the paediatrician to screen for any systemic anomalies, paediatric ophthalmologist to assess for visual potential and the oculoplastic surgeon for eyelid and socket rehabilitation. A stepwise algorithm can be followed for the management of these patients:

1. Expansion of lids/phimosis
2. Expansion of fornices
3. Expansion of bones

The mainstay of treatment is to give serially enlarging conformer which should be started in the first few weeks of life. They help in stretching the eyelids as well as the conjunctival fornices. Once the socket outgrows a particular sized conformer, it can be replaced with the next bigger sized one. Forniceal expansion can also be achieved with hydrogel hemispherical expanders which are placed in the conjunctival fornix followed by a tarsorrhaphy. The tarsorrhaphy is released after 2–3 months, and this can be followed by the placement of an acrylic conformer for further socket expansion [4, 7]. In an eye with microphthalmos, the eye can be preserved until orbital growth is complete unless it is diseased since it provides a stimulus for orbital growth and also gives better motility for the prosthesis [8]. Once the fornices are adequately expanded, the volume deficit can be corrected with orbital expanders—hard spherical implant (acrylic/silicon), inflatable soft orbital expanders, dermis fat grafts, hydrogel osmotic expanders or the recent integrated orbital tissue expanders [9–11]. The static spherical implants have the disadvantage of subjecting the child to repeated anaesthesia and surgeries to obtain orbital and facial symmetry. Although the inflatable soft tissue expanders are effective, the direction of expansion is unpredictable and can sometimes lead to conformer extrusion and pressure atrophy of surrounding tissues [5, 12, 13]. The hydrogel expanders come as either spheres or pellets. They are injected in their dry anhydrous state, and once placed, imbibe water and expand up to 30 times their volume (for spheres) and 10 times (for pellets). Once they reach equilibrium with surrounding structures, further expansion ceases and may need to be exchanged (for spheres) or require re-injections (for pellets). Moreover, potential adverse effects like migration, uncontrolled expansion, foreign body reaction and infection remain. Recently, Tse et al. have developed a new device called the integrated orbital tissue expander (OTE) which consists of an inflatable balloon attached to a titanium fixation plate [9–11]. The titanium plate can be fixed to lateral orbital rim with screws ensuring unidirectional expansion unlike other inflatable expanders. The OTE is also provided with an injection port through which a 30G needle connected to a 1 cc syringe can be inserted to inflate the expander. The port seals after removal of the needle. Thus, it eliminates the use of any conjunctival or soft tissue incision. It was also found that in addition to orbital growth stimulation, this device induced the growth of surrounding bones like the maxilla and zygoma and provided better eyebrow position, facial fullness and symmetry [11].

Acquired Socket Contracture

Krishna [3] in his study found that the socket contracture was most severe in cases of chemical injuries followed by panophthalmitis, perforated injuries, endophthalmitis, retinoblastoma and least in microphthalmos. Non placement of primary implant after evisceration/enucleation is also an important cause of socket contracture. Once socket contracture sets in, the first thing to do is to identify the cause of the contracture, and treat it accordingly. The two broad categories under which this can be discussed are:

1. Management of volume deficit
2. Management of deficient surface

1. Management of volume deficit—This can be corrected with the use of orbital implants. Primary volume replacement is preferred unless it is contraindicated as in cases of severe ocular trauma or infection (inhibiting closure of the wound) [14]. If not so, secondary implantation or a dermis fat graft should be considered. The various methods used for volume replacement for the anopthalmic socket are as follows:
    (a) Autologous implants
        • Dermis fat graft (DFG; Figs. 7.5, 7.6 and 7.7)—It provides for both volume and surface deficiency. It is taken from patient's own body tissue—gluteal region, anterior abdominal wall (non-hair bearing). The advantages of a DFG are as follows:
            – Nil chances of extrusion/migration
            – Replaces both volume and surface deficiency, so these are good for severely contracted sockets with severe forniceal shortening

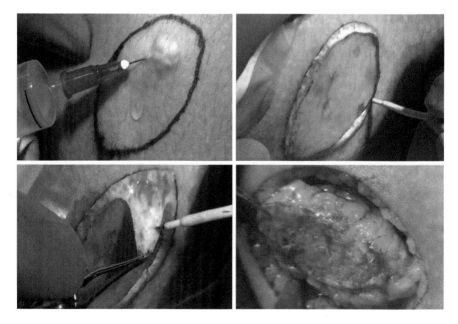

Fig. 7.5 Photographs showing steps of harvesting the dermis fat graft from the upper outer quadrant of the buttock

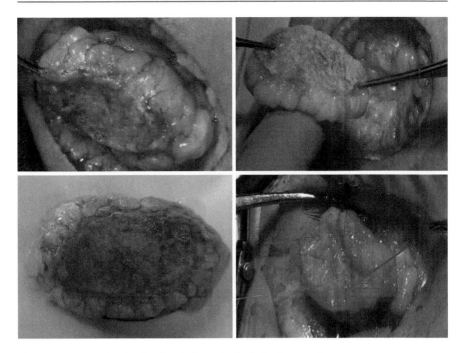

Fig. 7.6   Photographs showing dermis fat graft after being harvested

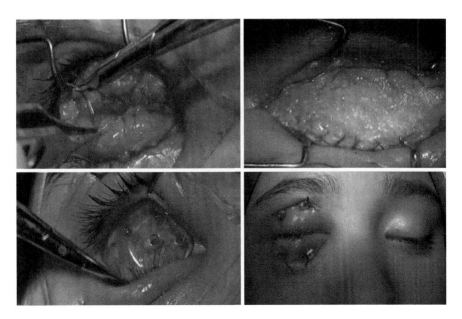

Fig. 7.7   Photographs showing steps of placement of DFG in the contracted socket with the dermis side facing up followed by suturing, fitting of conformer, fornix forming sutures and lid closure with temporary tarsorrhaphy

- Preferred for growing children as it has a tendency to expand with growth of the child
- Does not need a wrapping material for implantation

Some of the drawbacks of DFG are listed below:

- Graft can undergo central ulceration, necrosis and melt.
- Donor site morbidity.
- Can undergo fat atrophy and lead to suboptimal volume replacement or excessive fat proliferation if the patient gains weight.
- Chances of graft failure is high if the socket is ischemic/dry (post radiotherapy patients with repeated socket surgeries as the chance of bed vascularity is compromised).

(b) Synthetic orbital implants—The size of the implant to be placed can be calculated on the basis of the axial length of the other eye. If the implant is to be wrapped, 1 mm is subtracted from the axial length reading [15, 16]. After evisceration, these implants can be placed directly within the scleral coat and sutured in layers over it. But following enucleation, PMMA (polymethyl methacrylate) implants can be placed directly in the intraconal space or integrated implants need to be wrapped in materials such as sclera, dura, pericardium, fascia lata, temporalis fascia, alloderm and vicryl mesh to attach the extraocular muscles [17]. Depending on how the implant is connected to the overlying prosthesis, these can be divided into three types:

- Non-integrated: silicon or acrylic
- Semi-integrated: Allen implant, Iowa implant, Medpor quad implant
- Integrated: hydroxyapatite (HA)—natural coralline or synthetic
    o Porous polyethylene (Medpor)
    o Aluminium oxide (Bioceramic implants)
- Non-integrated (non-porous)

    These are spheres made of inert material like silicon or acrylic and have no connection with the overlying prosthesis as the anterior surface is fully covered by the overlying Tenon's and conjunctiva.

    They are inert and lack ingrowths of fibrovascular tissue and hence have higher rates of migration but lower chances of implant exposure. Using the myoconjunctival technique in enucleation, the motility of the custom ocular prosthesis over it can be increased. Non-integrated implants are implants of choice when an exchange of implant may be required later and are generally inexpensive.

    A 18 mm diameter, sphere typically gives a volume of 3.1 mL, while a 20 mm sphere gives a volume of 4.2 mL. The implant size should be customized to the particular individual [15–18].

- Semi-integrated

    They can be porous or non-porous.

    These implants remain buried under the conjunctiva and do not have a peg system. Instead they have a rough anterior surface which provides indirect coupling of the prosthesis resulting in better motility. However,

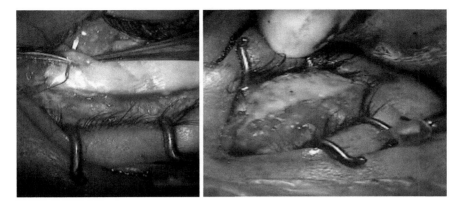

Fig. 7.8 Photographs showing use of oral mucus membrane graft in the management of mild socket contracture

the risk of exposure using them is significantly high. Examples are Allen Implant, Iowa Implant and Medpor Quad Implant.

- Integrated implants (porous implants)

  These implants have a regular system of interconnecting pores which allow fibrovascular ingrowth which reduces the chances of migration and extrusion of the implant.

  The time for fibrovascular ingrowth varies between 4 and 12 months [4] after which a motility peg can be inserted usually at 6 months to 1 year.

  The risk of thinning and erosion of the Tenon's and conjunctiva is very high and may be associated with formation of pyogenic granulomas or orbital infection.

  They are of following types:
  - Hydroxyapatite (HA)—natural coralline or synthetic
  - Porous polyethylene (Medpor)
  - Aluminium oxide (Bioceramic implants)

2. Management of deficient surface.
3. Grafts are used to increase the surface area.
   - Moist surface—mucous membrane graft (Fig. 7.8) from oral mucosa of cheeks/lips, hard palate, preputial skin and labial mucosa
   - Amniotic membrane graft
   - Dry surface—split thickness skin graft

Mild Socket Contracture

Mild contractures are associated with posterior lamella shortening causing vertical eyelashes and/or entropion. A tarsotomy and tarsal rotation may suffice to evert the lashes and rectify the entropion if that does not cause the depth of the fornices to reduce. The entropion correction can be planned in combination with mucous membrane grafts (MMG). Some patients have inadequate inferior forniceal space with adequate amount of conjunctiva. These patients have disinsertion of the inferior suspensory ligament of the fornix with associated anterior migration of inferior orbital fat. They form part of the anophthalmic socket syndrome. Such patients benefit from fornix forming sutures to reform the inferior fornix. A double armed 5-0 polyester/prolene suture is passed from fornix through the lower orbital rim periosteum and out on the skin surface where they are tied over bolsters and removed after 2–3 weeks.

If the patient has marked lower lid retraction associated with forniceal contraction, the posterior lamella may need to be lengthened with the placement of a spacer graft which may be autogenous, allogenous or synthetic.

Moderate Socket Contracture

A moderate socket contracture includes contracture of both the superior and inferior conjunctival fornices. The superior fornix even if shallow allows retention of the prosthesis though lid closure and prosthesis movement is compromised due to deficient forniceal depth. The goal of treatment in such cases is to allow for comfortable wear of prosthesis with reasonably good cosmesis [8]. This is achieved with the use of mucous membrane grafts (MMG) to make up for the deficient conjunctival surface.

The most common sites for MMG harvesting are the lip mucosa or the buccal mucosa.

Hard palate mucosal grafts may also be used and they have the advantage of less tissue contracture, but they have limited surface area available for harvesting. Amniotic membrane graft transplantation (AMT) has also been used for socket contracture. Its antifibroblastic, anti-inflammatory and growth promoting properties have long been known. A study done by Kumar et al. [19] found better patient comfort, lesser contracture and comparable retention of prosthesis in patients with mild to moderate socket contracture who underwent AMT when compared with those who underwent MMG. But AMT is a substrate graft, not a substitute graft like MMG. So it can be used only for mild to moderate contracture and not for severe contracture where there is gross deficiency of normal healthy conjunctiva.

Severe Socket Contracture

A DFG can be tried for severe socket contracture, but chances of graft atrophy due to poor vascularity remains. This can be combined with a temporalis muscle/fascial pedicled flap. This flap is based on the superficial temporal artery and will improve vascularity as well as increase the volume of the DFG when used in combination. In this procedure, a 25 mm wide pedicle of temporalis muscle with the epicranium is transposed through a bony defect created in lateral orbital wall into the orbit and sutured to the posterior Tenon's capsule and the periosteum medially [20]. The most common adverse effect seen is alopecia which may be transient or permanent. For very severe contracture, such as post radiation with almost no conjunctiva, microvascular radial forearm free flaps have been used with reasonable success and cosmesis [21]. Other flaps which have been used with encouraging results include thoracodorsal artery trilobed adiposal flap and retroauricular island flap [22, 23]. Complete excision of all lining tissue with permanent closure of eyelids is used as last resort for patients who have undergone multiple socket surgeries in the past with repeated failures. In these patients, placement of an immobile prosthesis which matches the other eye may offer a better option than any further surgeries [24]. Optical camouflage methods like use of tinted glasses, plus/minus power lenses and prisms have been used to improve the cosmesis.

Summary

The reconstruction of an anophthalmic socket especially after the development of contracture is challenging due to the increased risk of complications. Prevention is the key wherever possible. Meticulous surgical dissection and tailor-made selection of the ideal implant for each case is the tenet in the management of an anophthalmic socket. Socket reconstruction should be visualized as a team approach involving not just the oculoplastic surgeon but also the ocularist, the paediatrician, paediatric ophthalmologist and the maxillofacial plastic surgeon.

Disclosures None.

References

1. Bhattacharjee K, Bhattacharjee H, Kuri GK, Das JK, Dey D. Comparative analysis of use of porous orbital implant with mucus membrane graft and dermis fat graft as a primary procedure in reconstruction of severely contracted socket. Indian J Ophthalmol. 2014;62:145–53.
2. Gougelmann HP. The evolution of the ocular motility implant. Int Ophthalmol Clin. 1976;10:689–711.
3. Krishna G. Contracted sockets—I (aetiology and types). Indian J Ophthalmol. 1980;28(3):117–20.
4. Gundlach KKH, Gutoff RF, Hingst VHM, et al. Expansion of the socket and orbit for congenital clinical anophthalmia. Plast Reconstr Surg. 2005;116:1214–22.
5. Dunaway DJ, David DJ. Intraorbital tissue expansion in the management of congenital anophthalmos. Br J Plast Surg. 1996;49:529–35.
6. Sinclair D, Dangerfiled P. Nervous system. In: Sinclair D, Dangerfield P, editors. Human growth after birth. Oxford: Oxford University Press; 1998. p. 87.
7. Weise KG, Vogel M, Guthoff R, Gundlach K. Treatment of congenital anophthalmos with self-inflating polymer expanders: a new method. J Craniomaxillofac Surg. 1999;27:72–6.
8. Jordan DR, Klapper SR. Evaluation and management of the anophthalmic socket and socket reconstruction. In: Smith and Nesi's ophthalmic plastic and reconstructive surgery. 3rd ed. Berlin: Springer; 2012. p. 1131–73.

9. Tse DT. Inventor; University of Miami (Miami, FL) assignee. Integrated rigid fixation orbital expander. US patent 6,582,465 B2 June 2003.
10. Tse DT, Pinchuk L, Davis S. Evaluation of an integrated orbital tissue expander in an anophthalmic feline model. Am J Ophthalmol. 2007;143(2):317–27.
11. Tse DT, Abdulhafez M, Orozco MA, Tse JD, Azab AO, Pinchuk. Evaluation of an integrated orbital tissue expander in congenital anophthalmos: report of preliminary clinical experience. Am J Ophthalmol. 2011;15(3):470–82.
12. Tucker SM, Sapp N, Collin R. Orbital expansion of congenitally anophthalmic socket. Br J Ophthalmol. 1995;79:667–71.
13. Chen D, Heher K. Management of the anophthalmic socket in pediatric patients. Curr Opin Ophthalmol. 2004;15:449–53.
14. Leatherbarrow B. Oculoplastic surgery. 2nd ed. London: Informa; 2011.
15. Kaltreider SA. The ideal ocular prosthesis: analysis of prosthetic volume. Ophthal Plast Reconstr Surg. 2000;16:388–92.
16. Kaltreider SA, Lucarelli MJ. A simple algorithm for selection of implant size for enucleation and evisceration. Ophthal Plast Reconstr Surg. 2002;18:336–41.
17. Yoon JS, Lew H, Kim SJ, Lee SY. Exposure rate of hydroxyapatite orbital implants a 15-year experience of 802 cases. Ophthalmology. 2008;115(3):566–72.
18. Custer PL, Trinkaus KM. Volumetric determination of enucleation implant size. Am J Ophthalmol. 1999;128:489–94.
19. Kumar S, Sugandhi P, Arora A, Pandey PK. Amniotic membrane transplantation versus mucous membrane grafting in anophthalmic contracted socket. Orbit. 2006;25:195–203.
20. Bosnaik, et al. Temporalis muscle transfer: a vascular bed for autogenous dermis fat orbital implantation. Ophthalmology. 1985;92:292.
21. Li D, Jie Y, Liu H, Liu J, Zhu Z, Mao C. Reconstruction of anophthalmic orbits and contracted eye sockets with microvascular radial forearm free flaps. Ophthal Plast Reconstr Surg. 2008;24(2):94–7.
22. Koshima I, Narushima M, Mihara M, et al. Short pedicle thoracodorsal artery perforator (TAP) adiposal flap for three dimensional reconstruction of contracted orbital cavity. J Plast Reconstr Aesthet Surg. 2008;61:13–7.
23. Lopez-Arcas JM, Martin M, Gomez E, et al. The Guyuron retroauricular island flap for eyelid and eye socket reconstruction in children. Int J Oral Maxillofac Surg. 2009;38:744–50.
24. Rycroft BW. An operation for treatment of severe contraction of the eye socket. Br J Ophthalmol. 1962;46:21–6.

Targeted and Immune Therapy for Periocular and Orbital Malignancies

8

Oded Sagiv, Bashar Jaber, and Bita Esmaeli

Introduction

Periocular and orbital malignant tumors comprise a variety of neoplasms for which different treatment strategies may be appropriate. While the mainstay of treatment for most orbital tumors is surgical resection of the tumor, the recent use of targeted agents and immune-checkpoint inhibitors has contributed significantly to the management of patients with locally advanced, unresectable, or metastatic lesions. In this chapter, the current nonsurgical targeted biologic and immunotherapy treatment options are reviewed and possible future directions relevant to orbit and periocular cutaneous cancers are discussed.

Targeted Biologic Therapy

Targeted therapy drugs target specific molecules that are needed for tumor growth and carcinogenesis. This is different from traditional chemotherapy that affects all rapidly dividing cells. In recent years, several targeted drugs have been used to treat metastatic and locally advanced periorbital and orbital cutaneous cancers, specifically squamous cell carcinoma (SCC), basal cell carcinoma (BCC), and melanoma.

O. Sagiv · B. Esmaeli (✉)
Orbital Oncology and Ophthalmic Plastic Surgery, Department of Plastic Surgery,
The University of Texas MD Anderson Cancer Center, Houston, TX, USA
e-mail: besmaeli@mdanderson.org

B. Jaber
Orbital Oncology and Ophthalmic Plastic Surgery, Department of Plastic Surgery,
The University of Texas MD Anderson Cancer Center, Houston, TX, USA

St John Eye Hospital Group, Jerusalem, Israel
e-mail: Bashar.Jaber@sjeh.org

© Springer Nature Singapore Pte Ltd. 2019
A. Gupta, P. Tahiliani (eds.), *Orbit and Oculoplastics*, Current Practices in
Ophthalmology, https://doi.org/10.1007/978-981-13-8538-4_8

Sonic Hedgehog Inhibitors

Mutations that cause abnormal activation of the Sonic Hedgehog (SHH) pathway have been seen in several cancers, including sporadic BCC, patients with basal cell nevus syndrome (BCNS), and squamous cell carcinoma (SCC). SHH inhibitors block the activation of transcription factors of the SHH pathway by targeting the protein smoothened (smo), a key protein in SHH pathway.

(a) **Vismodegib:** Vismodegib (Erivedge, Genentech) was the first SHH inhibitor approved by the US FDA in 2012. It is given orally in a dose of 150 mg OD daily. It is approved for the treatment of locally advanced BCC that has recurred after surgery, metastatic BCC, and for patients who cannot undergo surgery or radiation therapy [1].
   Scientific evidence:
   - **Metastatic or locally advanced BCC:** Several major clinical trials have assessed the use of vismodegib for the treatment of metastatic or locally advanced BCC.
     - **ERIVANCE trial:** The investigators found that objective response rate (ORR) was 48.5% for metastatic BCC and 60.3% for locally advanced BCC. Median duration of response was 14.8 and 26.2 months, respectively. Median overall survival was 33.4 months in the metastatic BCC cohort and not estimable in the locally advanced BCC cohort [2].
     - **EAS trial:** ORR was 30.8% for metastatic BCC and 46.4% for a locally advanced BCC. Median duration of response was not assessed in this trial because of short duration of treatment [3].
     - **STEVIE trial:** This European trial reported an ORR of 37.9% for metastatic BCC and 66.7% for locally advanced BCC. Median duration of response was 10 months for metastatic BCC and 22.7 months for the locally advanced BCC [4].
     - **Pooled data:** A systematic review and pooled analysis of vismodegib therapy for locally advanced and metastatic BCC that included eight pooled articles with 704 clinically evaluable patients showed that the ORR in locally advanced BCC had a weighted average of 64.7%, and a complete response average of 31.1%. ORR for metastatic BCC was 33.6% and complete response average was 3.9%. Median duration of therapy was 35.8 weeks [5].
   - **Basal cell nevus syndrome:** We have experienced significant response to vismodegib therapy in two patients with periocular BCNS, both showed complete response over a prolonged period of treatment (19–38 months) [6]. In a large study of 41 patients with BCNS with lesions in various anatomic sites who were treated with vismodegib, 26 patients had a reduced rate of new surgically eligible BCCs compared with 15 patients randomly assigned to placebo [7].
   - **Locally advanced periocular BCC:** In the periocular area, a locally advanced disease may involve the orbit, sinuses or brain, and may necessitate orbital exenteration. Thus, neoadjuvant use of SHH inhibitors may be of particular interest.

- In a small series, response rate to vismodegib was 86% for locally advanced BCC, 100% for BCNS and 33% for metastatic BCC [6, 8, 9].
- There have been anecdotal reports of the combined use of SHH inhibitors with other treatments. One study of six patients found that treatment with SHH inhibitors, combined with radiation and mTOR inhibitors, for very large BCCs enabled a less-extensive resection at the definitive surgery.
- In another study, 15 patients with locally advanced periocular or orbital BCC, with mean treatment duration of 13 months, and mean follow-up of 36 months, ten (67%) patients showed complete response, three patients (20%) had a partial response while two (13%) had progressive disease following an initial response [10]. However, this study labeled complete response based only on clinical findings and not by a repeat surgical biopsy, and in fact, not all patients underwent surgery.
- We have published our experience of treating ten patients with locally advanced BCC who were not eligible for radiation therapy with vismodegib, four of whom had metastatic disease [8]. At the time of reporting the outcome, two patients had complete response, four patients had a partial response while disease of two patients had stabilized. The other two patients had disease progression: one patient progressed after 14 months of treatment with partial response and 3 months with no treatment, and one patient progressed after 16 months of treatment with stable disease and eventually died of his disease. The overall response rate for patients with non-metastatic locally advanced BCC was 86%. Five of these patients would have been treated with orbital exenteration as the surgical option for their tumor, but all were able to have an eye-sparing surgery eventually.

    These results, and the potential ocular toxicity expected from orbital radiation therapy, encouraged us to treat additional patients with locally advanced periocular BCC with vismodegib as a neoadjuvant agent with promising results. After the treatment was completed, all patients had an eye-sparing surgery with complete tumor removal and margins free of tumor (Fig. 8.1). Based on our findings, surgery seems to be warranted since nearly half (43%) of the patients with a complete clinical response were found to have residual tumor on pathological analysis of the surgical specimens (unpublished data, manuscript in preparation).

(b) *Sonidegib:* In 2015, sonidegib (Odomzo, Novartis), was approved by the FDA for locally advanced BCC that has recurred post-surgery or post-radiation, and for BCC, that is not amenable to surgery or radiation [11]. It is given orally at a dose of 200 mg daily.

Scientific evidence:

- **Bolt study:** In a 30-month analysis of the randomized Phase II Bolt study, for the efficacy of sonidegib, ORRs were 56.1% for locally advanced BCC and 7.7% for metastatic BCC. Median duration of response was 26.1 and

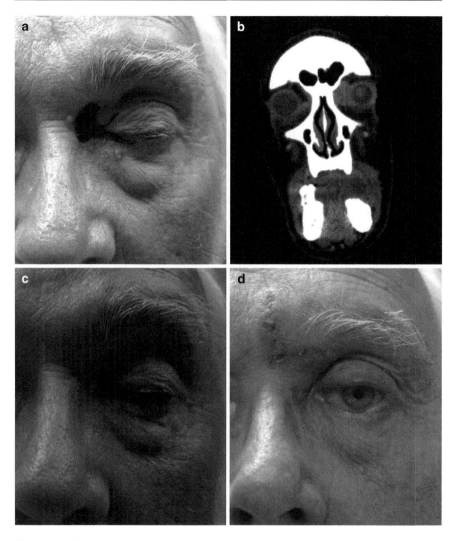

Fig. 8.1 A 61-year-old man who presented with a T4bN0M0 locally advanced nodular and infiltrative basal cell carcinoma involving the left lower and upper eyelids, and medial canthus (a). Imaging showed involvement of the left anterior orbit including the nasolacrimal duct (b). The patient was treated with neoadjuvant oral vismodegib 150 mg/day for 4 months with an excellent clinical response (c). He then underwent a wide local excision of the residual tumor with frozen section control of margins and reconstruction using a transposition myocutaneous flap (d). Final pathology found only fibrosis and inflammatory infiltrate with no evidence of tumor, making this a complete response to vismodegib. On follow-up of 2 months postoperatively, he is without evidence of disease

24.0 months, respectively. The 2-year overall survival rates were 93.2% and 69.3% for locally advanced and metastatic BCC, respectively [12].

- At the time of writing of this chapter, we were unable to find any reports on the efficacy of sonidegib for locally advanced periocular BCC.

Drug Resistance and Side Effects

Resistance to SHH inhibitors monotherapy, diagnosed clinically as tumor re-growth, has been reported in six patients (three of whom had BCNS) in a series of 28 patients within a mean time of 56 weeks [13]. Side effects from vismodegib treatment are common and have been reported in 98–100% of patients, but most are mild and tolerated by the patients.

The ERIVANCE study reported most (93%) of side effects to be of low to intermediate severity, that is Grade 1 (defined according to the Common Terminology Criteria for Adverse Events [CTCAE] version 4.03 as mild, asymptomatic or mild symptoms, clinical or diagnostic observations only, and intervention not indicated) or Grade 2 (defined as moderate, minimal, local, or noninvasive intervention indicated, and limiting age-appropriate instrumental activities of daily living) with only 7% being Grade 3 (defined as severe or medically significant but not immediately life-threatening, hospitalization, or prolongation of hospitalization indicated, disabling and limiting self-care activities of daily living) or higher [14, 15].

A recent review of nine studies confirmed that the majority of patients experienced only mild (Grade 1/2) side effects with the most common being muscle spasms (66.4%), alopecia (61.1%), dysgeusia (57.3%), weight loss (33.4%), amenorrhea (32.9%), and fatigue (20.1%) 0.5 calcium channel blockers (e.g., amlodipine 10 mg daily) was reported to help improve vismodegib-induced muscle spasms [16]. In our experience, most patients are able to tolerate long-term treatment. The oncologist can usually manage the side effects; and some side effects improve with a dose reduction to 5 times/week rather than daily.

Epidermal Growth Factor Receptor Antagonists

The understanding of the role of epidermal growth-factor receptor (EGFR) overexpression in squamous cell carcinoma led to the development of new therapeutic agents. Success has been reported in treating SCC of the head and neck region (HNSCC) [17]. The authors have previously shown overexpression of EGFR in conjunctival SCC as well [18].

(a) *Cetuximab:* Cetuximab (Erbitux, Lilly) is a monoclonal antibody EGFR antagonist that is US FDA-approved to treat locally or regionally advanced HNSCC in combination with radiation therapy or recurrent or metastatic HNSCC progressing after the treatment with platinum-based therapy [19].

Scientific evidence:

- In a multinational Phase III trial in patients with locally advanced HNSCC, the median duration of locoregional control was better in patients treated with cetuximab concurrent with radiation therapy compared with radiation therapy alone (24.4 vs. 14.9 months). Median overall survival was also improved (49 vs. 29.3 months), and a subsequent 5-year follow-up study demonstrated a superior overall survival rates (45.6% vs. 36.4%) [20].
- In another study of 36 patients with locally advanced HNSCC, a combination of cetuximab (induction followed by 7 weeks of weekly maintenance) and radiotherapy resulted in complete remission in 74% and partial remission in 17% [21].
- EXTREME trial: This trial showed that the addition of cetuximab to platinum-based combination chemotherapy in relapsing or metastatic HNSCC increased the overall survival from 7.4 to 10.1 months. It also improved the median progression free survival from 3.3 to 5.6 months [22].
- Another study found that cetuximab with docetaxel in 84 cases with recurrent or metastatic HNSCC resulted in partial remission in 11%, stable disease in 50%, and median overall survival of 6.7 months [23].

(b) *Erlotinib:* Erlotinib (Tarceva, Genentech) is a tyrosine kinase inhibitor EGFR antagonist that is FDA-approved for metastatic non-small cell lung cancer or pancreatic cancer, and has been studied as an off-label potential treatment for locally advanced HNSCC [17].

Scientific evidence:

- The use of erlotinib in locally advanced HNSCC as monotherapy and combined with either radiation or bevacizumab has demonstrated conflicting results [24–27].
- Soulieres et al. conducted a Phase II study in 115 patients with recurrent or metastatic HNSCC with an overall response rate of 4.3%. Disease was stabilized in 44 patients for a median duration of 16.1 weeks. Median progression-free survival was 9.6 weeks and median overall survival was 6 months [28].
- We reported our experience treating two patients with locally advanced periocular SCC invading the orbit with cetuximab, and erlotinib, with significant reduction in tumor size and improvement in quality of life [29]. Cetuximab in combination with platinum-based chemotherapy can also be used in the neoadjuvant setting to chemo-reduce large periorbital SCC and to reduce morbidity from surgery (Fig. 8.2).

Side Effects

Common adverse reactions with the use of EGFR inhibitors are skin rash, pruritus, nail changes, headaches, diarrhea, and infections. Some side effects may be correlated with better response to treatment: a Stage III study found overall survival significantly improved in patients who developed acne form rash of Grade 2 or higher

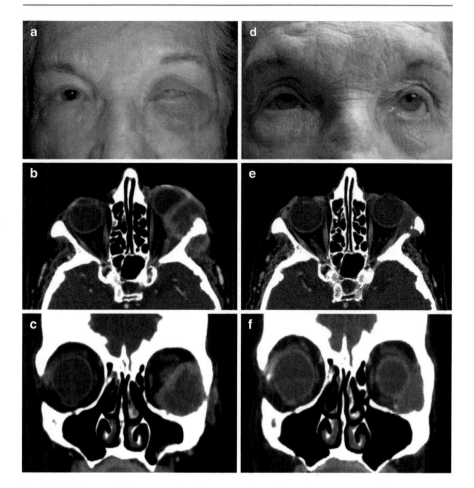

Fig. 8.2 A 89-year-old woman who had a squamous cell carcinoma removed from the lateral canthus elsewhere. A year later, she presented with left eye proptosis, periocular swelling and erythema, upper eyelid ptosis, and a palpable mass in the lateral canthus, lateral orbit, and temporal fossa (**a**). On examination, her visual acuity in the left eye was counting fingers and dilated fundus examination found choroidal striae. CT found a 3.1 × 3.2 × 4 cm mass that erodes through the inferolateral orbital wall and with an extraorbital extension of 4.2 × 2.3 × 2.5 cm (**b** and **c**). Work-up found metastatic disease to a left parotid lymph node which is confirmed with fine needle aspiration. The patient declined having an exenteration, parotidectomy, and lymph node dissection and was therefore treated with erlotinib 200 mg daily. She had a significant response to the treatment with a decrease in size of both the orbital lesion and the parotid lymph node within 3 months, resolution of orbital pain and improvement in visual acuity and motility, and this favorable clinical response was durable with no progression over noted at last follow-up 7 years after initial presentation(**d–f**)

compared with patients who experienced no rash or only Grade 1 [22]. From the ophthalmic perspective, EGFR inhibitors have been associated with uveitis, trichomegaly, corneal thinning and melting, and lower eyelid ectropion that was probably secondary [30].

BRAF Inhibitors

The BRAF gene, and its respective protein BRAF kinase, plays a key role in cell growth and proliferation. BRAF gene mutation was found in 50% of cutaneous melanomas, and the V600E mutation (substitution of valine for glutamate) was found in approximately 90% of these cases [31, 32]. The mutant protein causes abnormal activation of the MAPK signaling pathway, which results in persistent survival of affected cells and increased proliferation. Vemurafenib and dabrafenib are highly selective BRAF inhibitors, FDA-approved since 2011.

(a) *Vemurafenib:* Vemurafenib (Zelboraf, Genentech) is used for the treatment of metastatic or unresectable melanomas with positive V600E mutation [33].
(b) *Dabrafenib:* Dabrafenib (Tafinlar, Novartis) was FDA-approved in 2013 for the treatment of patients with metastatic or unresectable melanoma positive for V600E mutation. Dabrafenib was also approved for a combination treatment with trametinib (Mekinist, Novartis), a MEK inhibitor, for melanomas with BRAF V600E or V600K mutations [34, 35].
   Common side effects of BRAF inhibitors include fatigue, arthralgia and skin rash (the latter more common with vemurafenib) [32]. It has also been suggested that it increases the risk for epithelial proliferation and secondary skin cancers.

Scientific Evidence
Clinical trials have shown that successful inhibition of the MAPK signaling pathway by highly selective BRAF inhibitors in individuals with BRAF-mutated metastatic melanoma is associated with rapid therapeutic response in 50–80% of patients and prolonged progression-free survival of 6–10 months and overall survival of 16–20 months [36].

   Despite encouraging initial response, resistance to treatment has been developed in many cases after an average of 5–6 months of treatment. This is thought to happen from a bypass-activation of the MAPK pathway, frequently through abnormal activation of MEK. This results in re-growth of metastases that were previously in remission [37]. Several clinical trials have shown that patients with metastatic BRAF-mutated melanoma have a longer progression-free survival and overall survival when treated with combination therapy of BRAF and MEK inhibitors. The combination of vemurafenib and cobimetinib in the coBRIM study resulted in progression-free survival of 9.9 months and overall survival of 22.3 months, compared to 6.2 and 17.4 months with vemurafenib monotherapy [38, 39]. The combination of dabrafenib and

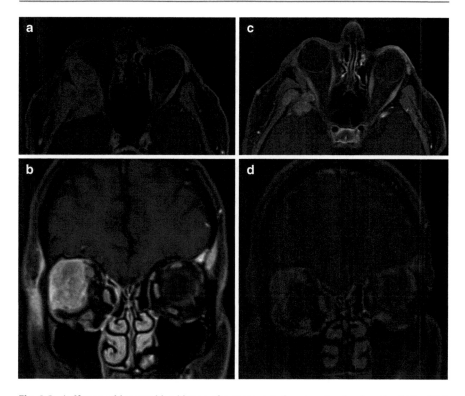

Fig. 8.3 A 63-year-old man with a history of cutaneous melanoma who developed a right orbital mass involving the right sphenoid wing and posterior orbit, compressing the optic nerve and causing severe optic neuropathy with reduced vision to head-motions and swelling of the optic disc (**a, b**). Histopathologic analysis of the biopsy found malignant melanoma positive for the BRAF V600E mutation. The patient was treated with trametinib 2 mg/day and dabrafenib 150 mg twice daily. After 2 months of treatment, his orbital metastasis had partial response to the treatment with considerable reduction in size and improvement in his symptoms (**c, d**). Unfortunately, he died 3 months later from progressive brain metastases

trametinib (COMBI-d study) resulted in progression-free survival of 11 months and overall survival of 25.1 months, compared to 8.8 and 18.7 months with dabrafenib monotherapy [40]. For these reasons, combination therapy with BRAF inhibitors and MEK inhibitors has largely replaced BRAF inhibitors monotherapy for patients with metastatic melanoma.

At the time of writing, we did not find reports of these drugs used for the treatment of eyelid melanomas specifically, but we have experienced positive responses in patients with cutaneous melanoma metastatic to the orbit (Fig. 8.3). The BRAF mutation was also found positive in 29–35% of conjunctival melanoma cases in retrospective pathologic studies [41, 42]. Dagi-Glass et al. have also reported positive response with dabrafenib and trametinib in a patient with a locally advanced and unresectable conjunctival melanoma [43].

Side Effects

Common side effects of BRAF inhibitors include arthralgia, alopecia, fatigue, photosensitivity reaction, nausea, pruritus and skin papillomas [33]. A recent meta-analysis of 1730 patients from five randomized controlled trials found that the combination therapy of BRAF inhibitors and MEK inhibitors significantly increased the incidence of certain adverse reactions such as hypertension, night sweats, pyrexia, chills, vomiting, and increased liver function tests, and ocular adverse reactions such as serous chorioretinopathy and retinal detachment [44]. In a meta-analysis of 7442 patients, BRAF inhibitors were also found to cause growth of cutaneous SCC in 12.5% of patients treated with BRAF inhibitors, compared with only 3% in patients treated with a combination of BRAF and MEK inhibitors [45]. We have previously reported our experience with patients who developed keratinocytic neoplasms of the eyelids while being treated with BRAF inhibitors, including invasive squamous cell carcinoma [46].

Immune Checkpoint Inhibitors

Programmed cell death protein 1 (PD-1) and cytotoxic T-lymphocyte antigen 4 (CTLA-4) are proteins found on the surface of activated T lymphocytes. When activated, they cause inhibition of proliferation of these cells. This inhibitory checkpoint is used by cancer cells to evade the immune system. Immune check-point inhibitors are a novel class of drugs that block these abnormally activated proteins, facilitating recognition of the cancerous cells by the host T lymphocytes, and enabling effective immune response against these cells. Currently there are several FDA-approved drugs of this class that can be considered for patients with unresectable or metastatic periocular tumors, such as locally advanced squamous carcinomas and melanoma.

(a) *Nivolumab:* Nivolumab (Opdivo, Bristol-Myers Squibb) was FDA-approved in 2014 for the treatment of patients with metastatic or unresectable melanoma and metastatic or recurrent squamous cell carcinoma of the head and neck (HNSCC) [47].

(b) *Pembrolizumab:* Pembrolizumab (Keytruda, Merck), FDA-approved since 2014, is indicated for the treatment of patients with metastatic melanoma and metastatic or recurrent HNSCC [48].

(c) *Ipilimumab:* Ipilimumab (Yervoy, Bristol-Myers Squibb) is a CTLA-4 inhibitor. It was FDA-approved in 2011 for the treatment of patients with metastatic or unresectable melanoma, as well as an adjuvant treatment for patients with melanoma with lymph node metastasis of more than 1 mm after total lymphadenectomy [49].

(d) *Avelumab:* Avelumab (BAVENCIO, EMD Serono), an anti-PD ligand-1 agent (anti-PD-L1), was FDA-approved in 2017 for the treatment of metastatic Merkel cell carcinoma [50].

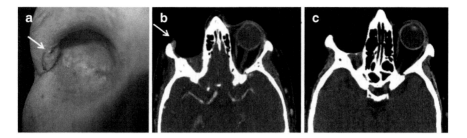

Fig. 8.4 (**a**) Clinical photo of patient no. 1 who developed local recurrence in the right orbital socket 1 year after undergoing orbital exenteration. She was found to have a 12 × 15 mm nodular mass along the lateral wall of the orbital socket (arrow) with adjacent areas of macroscopic ulceration (posterior to the nodule, not shown). (**b**) Computed tomography of the same patient form presentation, demonstrating a contrast-enhancing nodule at the anterior lateral orbital wall. (**c**) A computed tomography from 1 years later, after 3 months of treatment with nivolumab and 9 months of additional follow-up without treatment. There was no evidence for local recurrence at last follow-up

Scientific evidence:
- Improved survival was reported on large-scale trials in patients with unresectable or metastatic melanoma treated with ipilimumab [51, 52], pembrolizumab [53], and nivolumab [54–56].
- Different checkpoint inhibitors are also combined to maximize their synergistic effects. Anti-CTLA-4 acts during the priming phase, and anti-PD-1/PD-L1 are thought to act primarily during the effector phase in the tumor microenvironment.
- Studies have shown that combining ipilimumab with nivolumab or pembrolizumab is more effective, but also more toxic, than either single agent in both melanoma and non-small cell lung cancer [57, 58].
- Immunotherapy can also be combined effectively with chemotherapy, targeted therapy, and radiotherapy. The efficacy of chemotherapy combined with immunotherapy depends on the drug and on the relative timing of immunotherapy and chemotherapy [59].
- Positive response has also been reported to both nivolumab and pembrolizumab in patients with orbital metastasis from cutaneous melanoma, and in patients with eyelid and conjunctival melanoma with metastasis (Fig. 8.4) [60]. Preliminary positive results have also been noted for locally advanced recurrent SCC of the periocular region in response to immune checkpoint inhibitors.

Side effects of immune check point inhibitors

The side effects profile of the immune checkpoint inhibitors is different from that of traditional chemotherapy or targeted therapy since they are the result of activation of the immune system, following the release of the CTLA-4/PD-1 inhibition.

Common side effects include cutaneous rash, pruritus, colitis, autoimmune hepatitis, pneumonitis, and endocrinopathies such as hypophysitis or thyroid dysfunction. Neuropathy, myositis, and arthritis are less common but have been reported [61]. Ocular side effects include conjunctivitis, episcleritis, and uveitis. The authors have also experienced orbital inflammation (symptomatically similar to thyroid eye disease orbital inflammation) in a number of patients as a result of immune checkpoint therapy (unpublished data, manuscript in preparation). Serious side effects were more common with ipilimumab (10–15%) than with nivolumab or pembrolizumab (5%).

Conclusions

Advances in the field of medical oncology in recent years have revolutionized the treatment for patients with unresectable or metastatic cancers such as BCC, SCC, and melanoma. Promising results for both locally advanced and metastatic periocular tumor should encourage ophthalmologists and oculoplastic surgeons to implement these treatments for appropriate cases as described in this chapter.

The periocular region has unique characteristics and presents special considerations compared to other parts of the body as a locally advanced tumor may necessitate an orbital exenteration, and thus may not qualify as an "unresectable" tumor. However, given the degree of morbidity associated with orbital exenteration, targeted biologic and immunotherapy can be considered in patients with locally advanced periocular cancers who would otherwise need an orbital exenteration. Radiation therapy is also often associated with significant ocular toxicity in the periocular region thus further justifying the use of systemic targeted or immunotherapy as an attractive option instead. The neoadjuvant use of targeted biologic drugs and immunotherapy in patients with periocular locally advanced or metastatic cancer is currently evolving and needs more data.

References

1. US-FDA. FDA labeling information—ERIVEDGE. FDA website. 2012. https://www.access-data.fda.gov/drugsatfda_docs/label/2012/203388lbl.pdf.
2. Sekulic A, Migden MR, Basset-Seguin N, et al. Long-term safety and efficacy of vismodegib in patients with advanced basal cell carcinoma: final update of the pivotal ERIVANCE BCC study. BMC Cancer. 2017;17(1):332.
3. Chang AL, Solomon JA, Hainsworth JD, et al. Expanded access study of patients with advanced basal cell carcinoma treated with the Hedgehog pathway inhibitor, vismodegib. J Am Acad Dermatol. 2014;70(1):60–9.
4. Basset-Seguin N, Hauschild A, Grob JJ, et al. Vismodegib in patients with advanced basal cell carcinoma (STEVIE): a pre-planned interim analysis of an international, open-label trial. Lancet Oncol. 2015;16(6):729–36.
5. Jacobsen AA, Aldahan AS, Hughes OB, et al. Hedgehog pathway inhibitor therapy for locally advanced and metastatic basal cell carcinoma: a systematic review and pooled analysis of interventional studies. JAMA Dermatol. 2016;152(7):816–24.

6. Ozgur OK, Yin V, Chou E, et al. Hedgehog pathway inhibition for locally advanced periocular basal cell carcinoma and basal cell nevus syndrome. Am J Ophthalmol. 2015;160(2):220–227. e222.
7. Tang JY, Ally MS, Chanana AM, et al. Inhibition of the hedgehog pathway in patients with basal-cell nevus syndrome: final results from the multicentre, randomised, double-blind, placebo-controlled, phase 2 trial. Lancet Oncol. 2016;17(12):1720–31.
8. Yin VT, Esmaeli B. Targeting the hedgehog pathway for locally advanced and metastatic basal cell carcinoma. Curr Pharm Des. 2017;23(4):655–9.
9. Demirci H, Worden F, Nelson CC, et al. Efficacy of vismodegib (erivedge) for basal cell carcinoma involving the orbit and periocular area. Ophthal Plast Reconstr Surg. 2015;31(6):463–6.
10. Wong KY, Fife K, Lear JT, et al. Vismodegib for locally advanced periocular and orbital basal cell carcinoma: a review of 15 consecutive cases. Plast Reconstr Surg Glob Open. 2017;5(7):e1424.
11. US-FDA. FDA labeling information—ODOMZO. FDA website. 2015. https://www.access-data.fda.gov/drugsatfda_docs/label/2015/205266s000lbl.pdf.
12. Lear JT, Migden MR, Lewis KD, et al. Long-term efficacy and safety of sonidegib in patients with locally advanced and metastatic basal cell carcinoma: 30-month analysis of the randomized phase 2 BOLT study. J Eur Acad Dermatol Venereol. 2018;32(3):372–81.
13. Chang AL, Oro AE. Initial assessment of tumor regrowth after vismodegib in advanced Basal cell carcinoma. Arch Dermatol. 2012;148(11):1324–5.
14. Sekulic A, Migden MR, Oro AE, et al. Efficacy and safety of vismodegib in advanced basal-cell carcinoma. N Engl J Med. 2012;366(23):2171–9.
15. US_Department_of_Health_Human_Services. Common terminology criteria for adverse events (CTCAE) version 4.03, 2010. Bethesda, MD: National Institutes of Health, National Cancer Institute; 2016.
16. Ally MS, Tang JY, Lindgren J, et al. Effect of calcium channel blockade on vismodegib-induced muscle cramps. JAMA Dermatol. 2015;151(10):1132–4.
17. Moreira J, Tobias A, O'Brien MP, Agulnik M. Targeted therapy in head and neck cancer: an update on current clinical developments in epidermal growth factor receptor-targeted therapy and immunotherapies. Drugs. 2017;77(8):843–57.
18. Shepler TR, Prieto VG, Diba R, et al. Expression of the epidermal growth factor receptor in conjunctival squamous cell carcinoma. Ophthal Plast Reconstr Surg. 2006;22(2):113–5.
19. US-FDA. FDA labeling information—ERBITUX. FDA website. 2004. https://www.access-data.fda.gov/drugsatfda_docs/label/2009/125084s168lbl.pdf.
20. Bonner JA, Harari PM, Giralt J, et al. Radiotherapy plus cetuximab for locoregionally advanced head and neck cancer: 5-year survival data from a phase 3 randomised trial, and relation between cetuximab-induced rash and survival. Lancet Oncol. 2010;11(1):21–8.
21. Acevedo-Henao CM, Valette G, Miglierini P, et al. Radiotherapy combined with cetuximab for locally advanced head and neck cancer: results and toxicity. Cancer Radiother. 2012;16(7):601–3.
22. Vermorken JB, Mesia R, Rivera F, et al. Platinum-based chemotherapy plus cetuximab in head and neck cancer. N Engl J Med. 2008;359(11):1116–27.
23. Knoedler M, Gauler TC, Gruenwald V, et al. Phase II study of cetuximab in combination with docetaxel in patients with recurrent and/or metastatic squamous cell carcinoma of the head and neck after platinum-containing therapy: a multicenter study of the Arbeitsgemeinschaft Internistische Onkologie. Oncology. 2013;84(5):284–9.
24. Thomas F, Rochaix P, Benlyazid A, et al. Pilot study of neoadjuvant treatment with erlotinib in nonmetastatic head and neck squamous cell carcinoma. Clin Cancer Res. 2007;13(23):7086–92.
25. Herchenhorn D, Dias FL, Viegas CM, et al. Phase I/II study of erlotinib combined with cisplatin and radiotherapy in patients with locally advanced squamous cell carcinoma of the head and neck. Int J Radiat Oncol Biol Phys. 2010;78(3):696–702.
26. Hainsworth JD, Spigel DR, Greco FA, et al. Combined modality treatment with chemotherapy, radiation therapy, bevacizumab, and erlotinib in patients with locally advanced squamous

carcinoma of the head and neck: a phase II trial of the Sarah Cannon oncology research consortium. Cancer J (Sudbury, Mass). 2011;17(5):267–72.

27. Martins RG, Parvathaneni U, Bauman JE, et al. Cisplatin and radiotherapy with or without erlotinib in locally advanced squamous cell carcinoma of the head and neck: a randomized phase II trial. J Clin Oncol. 2013;31(11):1415–21.

28. Soulieres D, Senzer NN, Vokes EE, et al. Multicenter phase II study of erlotinib, an oral epidermal growth factor receptor tyrosine kinase inhibitor, in patients with recurrent or metastatic squamous cell cancer of the head and neck. J Clin Oncol. 2004;22(1):77–85.

29. El-Sawy T, Sabichi AL, Myers JN, et al. Epidermal growth factor receptor inhibitors for treatment of orbital squamous cell carcinoma. Arch Ophthalmol. 2012;130(12):1608–11.

30. Saint-Jean A, Sainz de la Maza M, Morral M, et al. Ocular adverse events of systemic inhibitors of the epidermal growth factor receptor: report of 5 cases. Ophthalmology. 2012;119(9):1798–802.

31. Chapman PB, Hauschild A, Robert C, et al. Improved survival with vemurafenib in melanoma with BRAF V600E mutation. N Engl J Med. 2011;364(26):2507–16.

32. Cosgarea I, Ritter C, Becker JC, et al. Update on the clinical use of kinase inhibitors in melanoma. J Dtsch Dermatol Ges. 2017;15(9):887–93.

33. US-FDA. FDA labeling information—ZELBORAF. FDA website. 2011. https://www.accessdata.fda.gov/drugsatfda_docs/label/2017/202429s012lbl.pdf.

34. US-FDA. FDA labeling information—TAFLINAR. FDA website. 2013. https://www.accessdata.fda.gov/drugsatfda_docs/label/2014/202806s002lbl.pdf.

35. US-FDA. FDA labeling information—MEKINIST. FDA website. 2013. https://www.accessdata.fda.gov/drugsatfda_docs/label/2014/204114s001lbl.pdf.

36. McArthur GA, Chapman PB, Robert C, et al. Safety and efficacy of vemurafenib in BRAF(V600E) and BRAF(V600K) mutation-positive melanoma (BRIM-3): extended follow-up of a phase 3, randomised, open-label study. Lancet Oncol. 2014;15(3):323–32.

37. Johannessen CM, Boehm JS, Kim SY, et al. COT drives resistance to RAF inhibition through MAP kinase pathway reactivation. Nature. 2010;468(7326):968–72.

38. Ascierto PA, McArthur GA, Dreno B, et al. Cobimetinib combined with vemurafenib in advanced BRAF(V600)-mutant melanoma (coBRIM): updated efficacy results from a randomised, double-blind, phase 3 trial. Lancet Oncol. 2016;17(9):1248–60.

39. Flaherty KT, Infante JR, Daud A, et al. Combined BRAF and MEK inhibition in melanoma with BRAF V600 mutations. N Engl J Med. 2012;367(18):1694–703.

40. Long GV, Stroyakovskiy D, Gogas H, et al. Dabrafenib and trametinib versus dabrafenib and placebo for Val600 BRAF-mutant melanoma: a multicentre, double-blind, phase 3 randomised controlled trial. Lancet. 2015;386(9992):444–51.

41. Larsen AC, Dahl C, Dahmcke CM, et al. BRAF mutations in conjunctival melanoma: investigation of incidence, clinicopathological features, prognosis and paired premalignant lesions. Acta Ophthalmol. 2016;94(5):463–70.

42. Griewank KG, Westekemper H, Murali R, et al. Conjunctival melanomas harbor BRAF and NRAS mutations and copy number changes similar to cutaneous and mucosal melanomas. Clin Cancer Res. 2013;19(12):3143–52.

43. Dagi Glass LR, Lawrence DP, Jakobiec FA, Freitag SK. Conjunctival melanoma responsive to combined systemic BRAF/MEK inhibitors. Ophthal Plast Reconstr Surg. 2017;33(5):e114–6.

44. Liu M, Yang X, Liu J, et al. Efficacy and safety of BRAF inhibition alone versus combined BRAF and MEK inhibition in melanoma: a meta-analysis of randomized controlled trials. Oncotarget. 2017;8(19):32258–69.

45. Peng L, Wang Y, Hong Y, et al. Incidence and relative risk of cutaneous squamous cell carcinoma with single-agent BRAF inhibitor and dual BRAF/MEK inhibitors in cancer patients: a meta-analysis. Oncotarget. 2017;8(47):83280–91.

46. Yin VT, Wiraszka TA, Tetzlaff M, et al. Cutaneous eyelid neoplasms as a toxicity of vemurafenib therapy. Ophthal Plast Reconstr Surg. 2015;31(4):e112–5.

47. US-FDA. FDA labeling information—OPDIVO. FDA website. 2017. https://www.accessdata.fda.gov/drugsatfda_docs/label/2017/125554s024lbl.pdf.

48. US-FDA. FDA labeling information—KEYTRUDA. FDA website. 2017. https://www.access-data.fda.gov/drugsatfda_docs/label/2017/125514s015lbl.pdf.
49. US-FDA. FDA labeling information—YERVOY. FDA website. 2015. https://www.accessdata.fda.gov/drugsatfda_docs/label/2015/125377s074lbl.pdf.
50. US-FDA. FDA labeling information—BAVENCIO. FDA website. 2017. https://www.access-data.fda.gov/drugsatfda_docs/label/2017/761049s000lbl.pdf.
51. Schadendorf D, Hodi FS, Robert C, et al. Pooled analysis of long-term survival data from phase II and phase III trials of ipilimumab in unresectable or metastatic melanoma. J Clin Oncol. 2015;33(17):1889–94.
52. Hodi FS, O'Day SJ, McDermott DF, et al. Improved survival with ipilimumab in patients with metastatic melanoma. N Engl J Med. 2010;363(8):711–23.
53. Barone A, Hazarika M, Theoret MR, et al. FDA approval summary: pembrolizumab for the treatment of patients with unresectable or metastatic melanoma. Clin Cancer Res. 2017;23(19):5661–5.
54. Beaver JA, Theoret MR, Mushti S, et al. FDA approval of nivolumab for the first-line treatment of patients with BRAFV600 wild-type unresectable or metastatic melanoma. Clin Cancer Res. 2017;23(14):3479–83.
55. Larkin J, Chiarion-Sileni V, Gonzalez R, et al. Combined nivolumab and ipilimumab or monotherapy in untreated melanoma. N Engl J Med. 2015;373(1):23–34.
56. Hazarika M, Chuk MK, Theoret MR, et al. U.S. FDA approval summary: nivolumab for treatment of unresectable or metastatic melanoma following progression on ipilimumab. Clin Cancer Res. 2017;23(14):3484–8.
57. Wolchok JD, Kluger H, Callahan MK, et al. Nivolumab plus ipilimumab in advanced melanoma. N Engl J Med. 2013;369(2):122–33.
58. Postow MA, Chesney J, Pavlick AC, et al. Nivolumab and ipilimumab versus ipilimumab in untreated melanoma. N Engl J Med. 2015;372(21):2006–17.
59. Emens LA, Middleton G. The interplay of immunotherapy and chemotherapy: harnessing potential synergies. Cancer Immunol Res. 2015;3(5):436–43.
60. Ford J, Thuro BA, Thakar S, et al. Immune checkpoint inhibitors for treatment of metastatic melanoma of the orbit and ocular adnexa. Ophthal Plast Reconstr Surg. 2017;33(4):e82–5.
61. Emens LA, Ascierto PA, Darcy PK, et al. Cancer immunotherapy: opportunities and challenges in the rapidly evolving clinical landscape. Eur J Cancer. 2017;81:116–29.

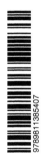